# Rhinology and Allergy for the Facial Plastic Surgeon

*Guest Editor*

STEPHANIE A. JOE, MD

# FACIAL PLASTIC SURGERY CLINICS OF NORTH AMERICA

www.facialplastic.theclinics.com

February 2012 • Volume 20 • Number 1

SAUNDERS an imprint of ELSEVIER, Inc.

**W.B. SAUNDERS COMPANY**
*A Division of Elsevier Inc.*

1600 John F. Kennedy Blvd., Suite 1800, Philadelphia, PA 19103-2899

http://www.theclinics.com

**FACIAL PLASTIC SURGERY CLINICS OF NORTH AMERICA Volume 20, Number 1**
**February 2012 ISSN 1064-7406, ISBN 978-1-4557-3858-8**

Editor: Joanne Husovski
Developmental Editor: Donald Mumford

*Facial Plastic Surgery Clinics of North America* (ISSN 1064-7406) is published quarterly by Elsevier Inc., 360 Park Avenue South, New York, NY 10010-1710. Months of issue are February, May, August, and November. Business and Editorial Offices: 1600 John F. Kennedy Blvd., Suite 1800, Philadelphia, PA 19103-2899. Periodicals postage paid at New York, NY, and additional mailing offices. Subscription prices are $359.00 per year (US individuals), $496.00 per year (US institutions), $409.00 per year (Canadian individuals), $594.00 per year (Canadian institutions), $489.00 per year (foreign individuals), $594.00 per year (foreign institutions), $170.00 per year (US students), and $237.00 per year (foreign students). Foreign air speed delivery is included in all *Clinics* subscription prices. All prices are subject to change without notice. POSTMASTER: Send address changes to *Facial Plastic Surgery Clinics*, Elsevier Health Sciences Division, Subscription Customer Service, 3251 Riverport Lane, Maryland Heights, MO 63043. **Customer service: 1-800-654-2452 (US and Canada); 1-314-447-8871 (outside US and Canada); Fax: 314-447-8029; E-mail:journalscustomerservice-usa@elsevier.com (for print support); journalsonline support-usa@elsevier.com (for online support).**

*Reprints.* For copies of 100 or more of articles in this publication, please contact the Commercial Reprints Department, Elsevier Inc., 360 Park Avenue South, New York, NY 10010-1710. Tel.: 212-633-3812; Fax: 212-462-1935; E-mail: reprints@elsevier.com.

*Facial Plastic Surgery Clinics of North America* is covered in *MEDLINE/PubMed* (*Index Medicus*).

Printed and bound by CPI Group (UK) Ltd, Croydon, CR0 4YY

Transferred to Digital Print 2012

# Contributors

## CONSULTING EDITOR

**J. REGAN THOMAS, MD, FACS**
Professor and Chairman, Department of
Otolaryngology, University of Illinois at
Chicago, Chicago, Illinois

## GUEST EDITOR

**STEPHANIE A. JOE, MD**
Associate Professor, Director, The Sinus &
Nasal Allergy Center; Co-Director, Skull Base
Surgery; Residency Program Director,
Department of Otolaryngology–Head and Neck
Surgery, University of Illinois at Chicago,
Chicago, Illinois

## AUTHORS

**TERAH J. ALLIS, MD**
Department of Otolaryngology–Head and Neck
Surgery, University of Nebraska Medical
Center, Omaha, Nebraska

**PETE S. BATRA, MD, FACS**
Associate Professor and Co-Director,
Comprehensive Skull Base Program,
Department of Otolaryngology–Head and Neck
Surgery, University of Texas Southwestern
Medical Center, Dallas, Texas

**SETH M. BROWN, MD, MDA, FACS**
Assistant Clinical Professor, Department of
Surgery, Division of Otolaryngology, University
of Connecticut School of Medicine,
Farmington, Connecticut

**PATRICK J. BYRNE, MD, FACS**
Associate Professor, Division of Facial Plastic
and Reconstructive Surgery, Departments of
Otolaryngology–Head and Neck Surgery and
Dermatology, Johns Hopkins Medical
Institutions, Baltimore, Maryland

**MOHAMAD CHAABAN, MD**
Department of Surgery, Section of
Otolaryngology–Head and Neck Surgery,
University of Chicago Medical Center,
Chicago, Illinois

**JASON Y.K. CHAN, MBBS**
Resident, Department of Otolaryngology–Head
and Neck Surgery, Johns Hopkins Medical
Institutions, Baltimore, Maryland

**JACQUELYNNE P. COREY, MD**
Department of Surgery, Section of
Otolaryngology–Head and Neck Surgery,
University of Chicago Medical Center,
Chicago, Illinois

**STEVEN MARC DAINES, MD**
Resident Physician, Division of
Otolaryngology–Head and Neck Surgery,
University of Utah School of Medicine,
Salt Lake City, Utah

**ANDREW J. HELLER, MD**
Chief, Section of Otolaryngology–Head and Neck Surgery, McGuire Veterans Affairs Medical Center; Clinical Associate Professor, Department of Otolaryngology–Head and Neck Surgery, Virginia Commonwealth University, Richmond, Virginia

**STEPHANIE A. JOE, MD**
Associate Professor, Director, The Sinus & Nasal Allergy Center; Co-Director, Skull Base Surgery; Residency Program Director, Department of Otolaryngology–Head and Neck Surgery, University of Illinois at Chicago, Chicago, Illinois

**JOHN H. KROUSE, MD, PhD**
Professor and Chairman, Department of Otolaryngology–Head and Neck Surgery, Temple University School of Medicine, Philadelphia, Pennsylvania

**DONALD A. LEOPOLD, MD, FACS**
Department of Otolaryngology–Head and Neck Surgery, University of Nebraska Medical Center, Omaha, Nebraska

**TODD A. LOEHRL, MD**
Professor and Chief of Rhinology/Sinus Surgery, Department of Otolaryngology and Communication Sciences, Zablocki VA Medical Center, Medical College of Wisconsin, Milwaukee, Wisconsin

**R. PETER MANES, MD**
Assistant Professor, Section of Otolaryngology–Head and Neck Surgery, Department of Surgery, Yale University School of Medicine, New Haven, Connecticut

**JAMES W. MIMS, MD**
Assistant Professor of Otolaryngology, Department of Otolaryngology, Wake Forest School of Medicine, Winston-Salem, North Carolina

**RICHARD R. ORLANDI, MD**
Associate Professor, Division of Otolaryngology–Head and Neck Surgery, University of Utah School of Medicine, Salt Lake City, Utah

**DOUGLAS D. REH, MD**
Assistant Professor, Department of Otolaryngology–Head and Neck Surgery, Johns Hopkins Medical Institutions, Baltimore, Maryland

**CORRIE E. ROEHM, MD**
Resident Physician, Department of Surgery, Division of Otolaryngology, University of Connecticut School of Medicine, Farmington, Connecticut

**BELACHEW TESSEMA, MD**
Assistant Clinical Professor, Department of Surgery, Division of Otolaryngology, University of Connecticut School of Medicine, Farmington, Connecticut

# Contents

This article defines chronic rhinosinusitis (CRS) and shares contemporary principles for its diagnosis and management, focusing on practical considerations for rhinoplasty surgeons. Nasal obstruction, the most common symptom of CRS, is frequently the chief complaint of patients seeking functional rhinoplasty surgery. Because correcting sites of anatomic obstruction to nasal airflow alone is unlikely to adequately treat CRS, rhinoplasty surgeons must have a firm understanding of the origin, diagnosis, and management of this disease process. With no single cause identified, CRS is likely an umbrella diagnosis or syndrome encompassing numerous causative factors, with the common end point of chronic sinonasal inflammation.

Familiarity with the diagnosis and management of allergic rhinitis is important for physicians concerned with the nasal airway. Allergic rhinitis is a common and manageable condition that may cause persistent or intermittent symptoms that vary as to duration and severity. Allergic rhinitis impairs quality of life, sleep, school performance, and productivity on a scale that compares with other chronic diseases. Diagnosis is primarily clinical, but supported by allergy testing. Therapeutic options for allergic rhinitis include pharmacotherapy, environmental control, and immunotherapy. More recently, a role for sublingual immunotherapy and turbinate reduction has been reported.

This article reviews a uniform way to describe nonallergic rhinitis in its various forms. The insights into its pathophysiology are briefly reviewed. A classification scheme for the different forms is provided. This is followed by descriptions of the diagnosis, evaluation, and management of nonallergic rhinitis.

The two most common allergic skin diseases in the world are often the least familiar to practicing surgeons: atopic dermatitis and contact dermatitis. When unrecognized, these disorders can cause great discomfort and decreased quality of life. This is only made worse by a surgical procedure which can exacerbate the disease process. Through proper recognition, management, and peri-surgical prophylaxis flares of these diseases can be avoided, leading to decreased morbidity and improved patient satisfaction. This article summarizes the pathophysiology and management of both atopic and contact dermatitis, with attention to implications for the surgeon.

Historically concurrent FESS/rhinoplasty was avoided due to concerns of increased risk of complication. Recent studies have shown that FESS/rhinoplasty can be performed simultaneously with good outcomes and no significant increase in complications. A thorough and effective approach to the patient with sinonasal obstruction requires attention to aesthetic, functional, and inflammatory issues. Medical treatment is an important adjuvant to surgery in order to optimize outcomes by improving patient symptoms long-term. Surgery for these patients should be performed in a careful, stepwise approach to address the nasal septum, inferior turbinates, paranasal sinuses, and external nasal structures.

The upper and lower respiratory tracts function as an interdependent physiologic mechanism, and stimuli that trigger pathophysiologic changes in one portion of the airway can provoke similar changes throughout the airway. The unified airway model acknowledges these shared airway features, suggesting the importance of comprehensive evaluation of patients with any respiratory symptoms. Two areas are of specific importance to the septoplasty/rhinoplasty surgeon: (1) preoperative evaluation of the patient with rhinitis undergoing nasal surgery, and (2) perioperative and postoperative management of the nose. Management of potential cardiopulmonary risks among susceptible individuals is vital in the perioperative management of these patients.

Concerns for the cosmetic surgeon regarding allergic rhinoconjunctivitis and rhinosinusitis include diagnosis, treatment, and assessment of the disease and whether or not the timing or outcome of cosmetic procedures will be affected. In this article, the pharmacotherapy of allergic and nonallergic rhinoconjunctivitis and rhinosinusitis is discussed with emphasis on intranasal steroids, antihistamines, and antibiotics.

Complementary and alternative medicine (CAM) includes treatments from traditional Chinese medicine, homeopathy, naturopathy, herbal medicine, Ayurvedic medicine, mind-body medicine, chiropractic or osteopathic manipulations, and massage. More than 40% of patients in the United States use CAM, with 17% of CAM use related to otolaryngology diagnoses, but nearly half of CAM users do not communicate their use of these medications to their physicians. Perioperative risk of bleeding is a particular concern in surgical specialties, and knowledge of these therapies and their potential adverse effects is critical.

Extraesophageal reflux has been implicated in many disorders affecting the upper airway. This article reviews the recent literature regarding the relationship of refractory chronic rhinosinusitis with extraesophageal reflux. Recent studies have shown that patients with refractory chronic rhinosinusitis have an increased prevalence of extraesophageal reflux. An association may exist between gastroesophageal reflux and rhinosinusitis, especially in individuals with medically and surgically refractory disease. These studies have a poor level of evidence and data supporting causation are lacking. However, evaluation and treatment should be considered in patients with chronic rhinosinusitis, especially in those with refractory disease.

Chronic rhinosinusitis (CRS) is a prevalent health care problem that may be commonly encountered in patients desiring aesthetic or reconstructive rhinoplasty. The purpose of this article is to review the common bacterial pathogens associated with CRS, as well as patterns of bacterial resistance in this patient subset. Close understanding of microbial pathogens involved in CRS and their associated resistance patterns will guide facial plastic surgeons in optimally managing this important potential comorbidity, and in turn positively influence the outcome of rhinoplasty.

Olfaction and taste promote satisfaction and protection in daily life. The astute facial plastic surgeon recognizes the importance of a baseline smell test to document the patients' olfactory status before surgery. After surgery, the surgeon must be alert to the possible mechanisms of hyposmia and anosmia and the pertinent treatment strategies. The surgeon must also understand the importance of counseling the patient and family regarding the cause of the dysfunction and the proper treatments. This article updates the facial plastic surgeon on the importance of smell and taste and associated disorders with a current review of the literature.

# Facial Plastic Surgery Clinics of North America

**THE CLINICS ARE NOW AVAILABLE ONLINE!**

Access your subscription at:
**www.theclinics.com**

# Rhinoplasty in Light of Sinonasal Issues

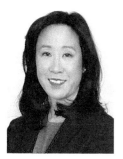

Stephanie A. Joe, MD
*Guest Editor*

I am honored to have been chosen to guest edit another issue of *Facial Plastic Surgery Clinics of North America*. This is a follow-up to the prior issue, "Rhinology for the Rhinoplasty Surgeon," published in 2004. Once again, I believe this issue represents the ideal blend of my background in both rhinology and facial plastic surgery and highlights the current topics facing the rhinoplasty surgeon.

The rhinoplasty surgeon must be aware of the possible sinonasal problems that may be present when discussing potential reconstructive or cosmetic nasal surgery with her or his patients. The presence of allergic rhinitis, nonallergic rhinitis, and/or chronic rhinosinusitis can affect the patients' perception of their nasal symptoms. Patients can suffer from skin-related sequelae to varying degrees. Familiarity with the smell and taste disorders provides rhinoplasty surgeons with additional information for the overall management of their patients. Resistant infections are a growing problem for all physicians.

Furthermore, surgical outcomes can be affected by the chronic inflammation associated with many of these conditions. With this in mind, I have included articles addressing the constantly evolving treatments for sinonasal disorders. There is one article on the current thinking on contemporaneous sinus surgery and rhinoplasty. There are articles on the role of conventional pharmacology and alternative medicine in rhinology. Lower airway problems and reflux may be uncovered during the evaluation for surgery and also may affect the management of sinonasal complaints.

The authors of this issue practice otolaryngology in a variety of disciplines—facial plastic surgery, rhinology, and otolaryngic allergy. I wish to thank them for their insightful contributions. I hope that this issue serves as a reference for all rhinoplasty surgeons and stimulates a continued dialogue between all otolaryngologists.

Stephanie A. Joe, MD
Department of Otolaryngology–Head
and Neck Surgery (MC 648)
University of Illinois at Chicago
1855 West Taylor Street, Room 2.42
Chicago, IL 60612, USA

E-mail address:
sjoe@uic.edu

Facial Plast Surg Clin N Am 20 (2012) ix
doi:10.1016/j.fsc.2011.10.012

# Chronic Rhinosinusitis

Steven Marc Daines, MD*, Richard R. Orlandi, MD

## KEYWORDS

- Chronic rhinosinusitis • Rhinoplasty
- Sinonasal inflammation • Surgery

---

**Key Points**

- Nasal obstruction, a common complaint of patients seeking functional rhinoplasty, is the most common symptom of chronic rhinosinusitis (CRS).
- CRS is an inflammatory process affecting the nose and paranasal sinuses that lacks a single clear origin.
- Treatment of CRS usually requires a multipronged approach incorporating nasal saline irrigations, topical steroids, management of comorbid conditions, and surgery in refractory cases.

---

Chronic rhinosinusitis (CRS), a disease characterized by symptomatic chronic inflammation of sinonasal mucosa, is estimated to affect 14% of the adult U.S. population.[1] CRS has been shown to affect a patient's quality of life similar to debilitating chronic medical conditions, such as congestive heart failure, chronic obstructive pulmonary disease, angina, and back pain.[2] The treatment of CRS accounts for a significant portion of health care use in the United States, with annual health care costs ranging from $4.3 to $5.8 billion[3] and an estimated 257,000 patients undergoing surgery for refractory CRS annually.[4] Nasal obstruction, the most common symptom of CRS, is also frequently the chief complaint of patients seeking functional rhinoplasty surgery.[5] Because correcting sites of anatomic obstruction to nasal airflow alone is unlikely to adequately treat CRS, rhinoplasty surgeons must have a firm understanding of the origin, diagnosis, and management of this disease process. To date, a single underlying cause for this disorder has not been identified. More appropriately, CRS is likely an umbrella diagnosis or syndrome encompassing numerous causative factors, with the common end point of chronic sinonasal inflammation. This article defines chronic rhinosinusitis (CRS) and shares contemporary principles for its diagnosis and management, focusing on considerations of practical relevance for the rhinoplasty surgeon.

## CHRONIC RHINOSINUSITIS DEFINED

Rhinosinusitis is defined as inflammation of the nose and paranasal sinuses characterized by two or more symptoms, one of which must be nasal blockage/obstruction/congestion or nasal discharge, and another either facial pain/pressure or a reduced sense of smell. For accurate diagnosis, the patient must also show endoscopic evidence of inflammation, including polyps, mucopurulent discharge, or edema, or computed tomographic mucosal changes within the osteomeatal complex or sinuses. Although acute rhinosinusitis is defined by a symptomatic period of up to 4 weeks with an eventual complete resolution of symptoms, the duration of symptoms in CRS is greater than 12 weeks and patients are never entirely symptom-free.[6]

CRS can be further subdivided based on the presence or absence of nasal polyps. On a microscopic level, polyps are edematous structures consisting of loose connective tissue, glands, and inflammatory cells. The most abundant

---

Division of Otolaryngology–Head & Neck Surgery, University of Utah School of Medicine, 50 North Medical Drive, 3C120, Salt Lake City, UT 84132, USA
* Corresponding author.
E-mail address: dainesmd@gmail.com

Facial Plast Surg Clin N Am 20 (2012) 1–10
doi:10.1016/j.fsc.2011.10.001
1064-7406/12/$ – see front matter © 2012 Elsevier Inc. All rights reserved.

facialplastic.theclinics.com

inflammatory cell in polyp tissue is the eosinophil, which is activated and sustained by the cytokine interleukin 5 (IL-5).[7]

No clear evidence explains why polyps develop in some patients and not in others. The prevalence of nasal polyps in the general population is 4%,[8] whereas in patients with asthma the prevalence increases to between 7% and 15%.[9,10] Despite the similarities between allergic rhinitis and nasal polyposis, including watery rhinorrhea, mucosal swelling, and eosinophilia, nasal polyps are only found in 0.5% to 1.5% of patients with positive skin prick tests for common allergens.[10,11] An association clearly exists between nasal polyposis and aspirin sensitivity, as evidenced by Samter's Triad (aspirin sensitivity, nasal polyposis, and asthma), yet not all patients with aspirin sensitivity have nasal polyps and vice versa.

An additional variant of CRS called *allergic fungal rhinosinusitis* has been described by Bent and Kuhn[12] based on five criteria: (1) nasal polyposis, (2) allergic mucin, (3) CT scan findings consistent with CRS, (4) positive fungal histology or culture, and (5) type I hypersensitivity diagnosed through history, skin test, or serology. Ferguson[13] described a related entity called *eosinophilic mucin rhinosinusitis*, which shares many of the clinical and pathophysiologic features of allergic fungal sinusitis but lacks the presence of fungus as a key element.

Although CRS encompasses a broad spectrum of distinct entities with unique clinical and pathologic phenotypes, they have a basic underlying commonality: symptomatic long-standing inflammation in the nose and paranasal sinuses. These distinct subtypes should be identified early in the workup of patients with sinonasal complaints, because they may each require distinct treatment algorithms and respond differently to medical and surgical management.

## ORIGIN OF CHRONIC RHINOSINUSITIS

Rhinosinusitis is often erroneously considered a strictly infectious process. Instead, it should be considered a multifactorial inflammatory process affecting the contiguous mucous membranes of the nose and paranasal sinuses. Although infection may be present and worsen CRS, additional factors also play important roles in initiating and sustaining chronic inflammation in the nose and paranasal sinuses.[14–19]

### Allergy

A history of atopy may predispose a patient to developing CRS.[20] Researchers have theorized that the swelling of nasal mucous membranes that accompanies allergic rhinitis may result in sinus ostial narrowing or obstruction, which can compromise ventilation and lead to mucous retention and infection.[21] Furthermore, just as the upper and lower airways are believed to represent a unified system, the nose and paranasal sinuses are also believed to be a physiologic continuum, responding in concert to their environment rather than in isolation.[22]

Allergic markers seem to be more prevalent in patients with CRS. Benninger[23] reported that 54% of patients with CRS had atopy based on positive skin prick tests. Multiple studies have shown that 50% to 84% of patients undergoing sinus surgery have a high incidence of positive skin prick tests.[24–26]

Although only 0.5% to 4.5% of patients with allergic rhinitis have nasal polyps,[10,11] the presence of allergy in patients with nasal polyps ranges from 10% to as high as 64%.[27,28] Levels of total and specific IgE have been associated with eosinophilic infiltration in nasal polyps.[29] Multiple studies have implicated food allergy as having a role in nasal polyposis.[30,31]

Not all studies support the role of allergy in the pathogenesis of CRS. In one study, no increase was seen in the incidence of rhinosinusitis during the pollen season in pollen-sensitized patients.[32] However, despite the lack of clear causal evidence for the role of allergy in CRS, failure to address allergy in patients with CRS reduces the probability of surgical success.[33] Furthermore, in patients undergoing immunotherapy, those who experienced the most subjective benefit for immunotherapy were those with a history of rhinosinusitis.

### Asthma

Although asthma is not a true cause of CRS, rhinoplasty surgeons should be aware of the strong association between the two disease processes. The unified airway theory holds that allergic inflammation coexists in the upper and lower airways.[34] Although rhinosinusitis and asthma frequently occur in the same patients, their interrelationship is not well understood. Studies in children have shown improvements in asthma symptoms and asthma medication use after surgery for CRS in pediatric patients with both conditions.[35,36]

The sinuses of asthmatic patients have shown radiographic evidence of abnormal mucosa.[37,38] In one study, all patients with steroid-dependent asthma had abnormal mucosal changes on CT compared with 88% of patients with mild to moderate asthma.[39]

Wheezing is reported in 31% of patients with nasal polyps, and asthma is reported by 26% of patients with nasal polyps compared with 6% of controls.[40] Late-onset asthma is associated with the development of nasal polyps in 10% to 15% of patients.[10] Although nasal polyps are twice as prevalent in men as in women, the coexistence of nasal polyps and asthma is twice as common in women than in men.[41]

## Anatomic Factors

Several variations in sinonasal anatomy have been proposed to have a role in CRS, including concha bullosa, nasal septal deviation, and variations in the uncinate process.[42,43] Despite a solid mechanistic foundation for this theory, investigators in two separate studies found no correlation between CRS and bony anatomic variations in the nose.[44,45] Several studies show that the prevalence of anatomic variations is no more common in patients with CRS than in the general population.[18,19,46] However, in a systematic review of the literature on the role of septal deviation in CRS, multiple studies showed that increasing angles of septal deviation were associated with increasing prevalence of rhinosinusitis. Although the association of septal deviation and rhinosinusitis was statistically significant, the overall clinical effect was modest, with an odds ration of 1.47. In all studies that examined the laterality of rhinosinusitis associated with septal deviation, inflammation was present bilaterally.[43] Based on these studies, the presence of variant anatomic structures may alter sinus ventilation and contribute to ostial obstruction, but alone is not sufficient for the development of CRS.

## Fungus

The presence of fungi in the human sinonasal cavity has been established. The influence of fungi can range from benign colonization, to noninvasive fungus balls, to fulminant invasive disease in immunocompromised patients.[47] Over the past decade, considerable debate has surrounded the role of fungi in CRS. In 1999, investigators proposed that eosinophilic infiltration and fungi were present in the sinuses of most patients with CRS.[48] These findings were based on positive fungal cultures using a new culture technique. However, using the same culture technique, normal controls were found to have a similar percentage of positive fungal cultures, casting doubt on the causative role of fungi in CRS.[49] Although a wide variety of fungi have been identified in the sinuses of patients with CRS, the presence of fungi does not confirm an etiologic role in the disease process.[50] Studies have not shown systemic or topical antifungals to be of benefit to patients with CRS.[51]

## Osteitis

Patients with CRS characteristically display areas of increased bone density and irregular thickening on CT, a finding that may be a marker of chronic inflammation.[52] Researchers have proposed that bony thickening may be a sign of inflammation of the bone, which may serve to perpetuate inflammation of the overlying mucosa.[53] Studies in rabbits showed that inflammation spread through the Haversian canals, resulting in chronic osteomyelitis at sites distant from the primarily involved sinus.[54] The concept of osteitis may explain why a nidus of inflammation in one sinus can result in pansinusitis, and may also account for why CRS can be refractory to even the most aggressive forms of treatment.

## Biofilms

A biofilm is a layer of adherent microorganisms attached to a surface and encased in a self-produced polysaccharide matrix.[55] Bacteria growing in biofilms can be unusually fastidious, resistant to fluctuations in moisture, pH, and temperature, and refractory to antibiotic therapy.[56] Biofilms have been identified as playing a potential role in otitis media, chronic tonsillitis, and adenoiditis in children with CRS, and they have also been seen on the mucosal surface of patients with CRS and on frontal recess stents.[57–61] The presence of bacterial biofilms could account for the chronicity of sinus inflammation in certain patients and could explain why patients experience improvement while on antibiotic therapy but relapse after finishing the medication.[62]

The presence of biofilms in patients with CRS does not explain the role these entities play in the disease process. In a recent study of patients with CRS with nasal polyps undergoing sinus surgery, biofilms were seen in both the treatment and control groups, suggesting that these entities are likely not sufficient to cause CRS without other cofactors.[55] Further studies are needed to clarify whether biofilms are innocent bystanders, initiators of mucosal inflammation, or perpetuators of a disease process already set in motion by other factors.

## Superantigens

Superantigens are microbe-produced toxins that bypass the specificity of the immune response and therefore activate up to 30% of lymphocytes. They have been proposed to play a role in CRS, particularly in patients with nasal polyposis. In one study, 55% of patients with CRS with nasal polyps had toxin-producing *Staphylococcus aureus* in the nasal mucus adjacent to the polyps. Three different enterotoxins were isolated and the corresponding variable β region of the T-cell receptor was upregulated in the polyp lymphocytes. The investigators proposed that the upregulation of lymphocytes by superantigens may result in the production of several cytokines that are responsible for the massive upregulation of eosinophils, lymphocytes, and macrophages, the three most common inflammatory cells in nasal polyps.[63]

### Mucociliary Impairment

Normal mucociliary clearance plays an important role in preventing chronic inflammation through transporting particles and bacteria trapped in the mucous blanket toward the sinus ostia, into the nasal cavity, and ultimately into the esophagus. As mucociliary clearance fails, bacterial export ceases and sinus mucosa is left vulnerable to noxious bacterial byproducts. Patients with Kartagener syndrome and primary ciliary dyskinesia frequently experience CRS, as do patients with cystic fibrosis whose viscous mucous cannot be adequately cleared through normal ciliary activity. Secondary ciliary dyskinesia develops in patients with CRS and, although likely reversible, restoration of normal ciliary function can take considerable time.[64]

### Other Factors

Although cigarette smoking was found to be associated with a higher prevalence of CRS in Canada,[65] a Korean study did not support these findings.[66] Like many chronic medical conditions, low income has been associated with a higher prevalence of CRS.[65] *Helicobacter pylori* DNA has been identified in 11% to 33% of sinus samples of patients with CRS but not in controls, although a causal relationship has not been proven.[67,68] Direct nasopharyngeal reflux of gastric acid has been implicated in patients with CRS refractory to endoscopic sinus surgery.[69] Finally, iatrogenic factors, including creation of a surgical antrostomy separate from the natural maxillary sinus ostium, can lead to mucous recirculation and persistent symptoms of CRS.[70]

## SYMPTOMS OF CHRONIC RHINOSINUSITIS

The symptoms of rhinosinusitis are well-known to facial plastic surgeons trained in otolaryngology and to rhinoplasty surgeons of other specialties. Nasal symptoms include nasal blockage, congestion, and stuffiness, and nasal discharge and reduction or loss of smell. Other local symptoms can include facial pain or pressure and headache.[6] Alterations in the sense of smell are more common in patients with nasal polyps than in other patients with CRS.[71]

Patients with CRS also frequently experience distant and constitutional symptoms. These include irritation of the pharynx and larynx leading to sore throat, cough, and dysphonia, and general symptoms of malaise and fatigue. Acute rhinosinusitis and acute exacerbation of chronic rhinosinusitis tend to have more distinct and severe symptoms.[6]

## DIAGNOSIS OF CHRONIC RHINOSINUSITIS

Methods for diagnosing CRS are numerous and include a variety of questionnaires, endoscopic and imaging scoring systems, and esoteric tests of sinonasal physiology.[6] For most surgeons performing rhinoplasty on a routine basis, these methods may be impractical and overly time-consuming. The authors suggest a simplified approach for diagnosing patients with CRS during the initial rhinoplasty consultation, who can then be offered additional diagnostic workup and management by the consulting rhinoplasty surgeon or referred to a specialist with expertise in the management of CRS.

### History

Patients seeking functional rhinoplasty frequently complain of nasal obstruction. Further questioning should be directed at determining the laterality of the obstruction, and the exacerbating and mitigating factors, seasonal variations in symptoms, or other temporal relationships. The presence of nasal discharge and its character should also be ascertained. Facial pain and pressure are common symptoms of CRS, although they may also be symptoms of other neurologic disorders, including trigeminal neuralgia or migraine. Fluctuations in olfaction are also associated with CRS, and an olfactory history should be elicited from every patient.

### Physical Examination

Although anterior rhinoscopy alone is usually inadequate to completely assess the nasal cavity and middle meatus, it can provide useful information to the examiner who otherwise lacks endoscopic equipment. The overall degree of inflammation of the mucosa and the presence of gross purulence or polyps coming from the middle meatus can be assessed. Finally, anatomic variants can be accounted for, such as septal deviations and hypertrophic inferior turbinates, and other pathology can be discovered, such as synechiae, tumors, and septal perforations.

For surgeons with endoscopic capabilities in their offices, endoscopy can be an invaluable tool for diagnosing the presence and severity of CRS. The presence of polyps, edema, crusting, discharge, and scarring can be identified and quantified,[72] and photos or video can be captured for future reference or comparison. Endoscopy also allows the surgeon to evaluate the posterior portion of the nasal cavity, a region that is not visualized with anterior rhinoscopy, including the region of the sphenoethmoid recess and nasopharynx. Additional abnormalities may be encountered on a more thorough endoscopic evaluation that would otherwise be overlooked.

### Ancillary Studies

CT scanning is the preferred imaging modality to confirm the extent of sinonasal pathology and define the anatomy of the nose and paranasal sinuses.

From a practical standpoint, imaging studies rarely should be ordered by a surgeon evaluating a patient for rhinoplasty but should instead be left to the discretion of the physician who will be definitively diagnosing and managing the patient's suspected rhinosinusitis over the long term.

Although a history of allergic rhinitis may eventually lead practitioners to order allergy testing, this line of investigation would not typically be pursued during the initial consultation for functional rhinoplasty.

## MANAGEMENT OF CHRONIC RHINOSINUSITIS

Treatment of CRS usually requires a multipronged approach, with surgery being reserved for refractory cases or those associated with impending orbital or intracranial complications. Rhinoplasty surgeons must be familiar with the medical and surgical options for treating nasal obstruction and other symptoms related to chronic sinonasal inflammation, because the nose does not exist in a treatment vacuum.

### Topical Corticosteroids

Multiple studies have evaluated the efficacy of topical corticosteroids in the treatment of patients with CRS with nasal polyps.[73–75] Overall, the preponderance of evidence shows some symptomatic improvement with the use of topical steroid sprays in patients with CRS.[6]

The treatment of CRS with nasal polyps with topical corticosteroids has been studied extensively. Most studies have shown significant improvement in symptoms such as nasal obstruction, loss of smell, and rhinorrhea, and in objective measures of nasal physiologic function.[76–78] Despite the infrequent occurrence of minor nosebleeds in patients using intranasal steroids, biopsies have failed to show detrimental effects on the nasal mucosa with long-term use.[79] Effects on the hypothalamic-pituitary-adrenal axis have not been shown.[80]

### Oral Corticosteroids

No studies have examined the use of oral corticosteroids for the treatment of CRS without nasal polyps. In patients with CRS with nasal polyps, however, recent well-designed studies have shown improvements in nasal symptoms and objective measures such as rhinomanometry, MRI scores, endoscopic findings, and CT changes after 2 weeks of oral steroid therapy.[81,82] The use of systemic steroids must always be weighed, of course, against the well-known side effects of this class of medication, including psychiatric effects, changes in bone mineral density, cataracts and glaucoma, and growth retardation in children.[83]

### Oral Antibiotics

No placebo-controlled studies have evaluated the effects of short-term antibiotics in patients with CRS. Although available studies in the literature show improvement in symptoms in most patients after short-term treatment with oral antibiotics, the specific antibiotic used seems to be of less importance.[6]

Long-term low-dose treatment with macrolide antibiotics seems to be effective in treating CRS refractory to surgical or steroid treatment.[84] Multiple explanations have been offered, but the definitive mechanism for the efficacy of macrolides in improving chronic inflammation is still unknown. Despite studies that seem to suggest a role for macrolides in CRS, treatment of refractory CRS with long-term low-dose macrolide therapy has yet to be supported by prospective placebo-controlled studies.

Side effects of antibiotics include allergic reactions, gastrointestinal symptoms, and other more rare but severe effects, such as damage to the bone marrow or other major organs. The development of antibiotic resistance is a global public health consideration that must also be recognized.

## Topical Antibiotics

A randomized double-blind trial of tobramycin-saline solution versus saline alone delivered through a nebulizer did not show a significant difference between the groups after 4 weeks of therapy.[85] Scheinberg and Otsuji[86] found an 82.9% response rate after treatment with aerosolized antibiotics for 3 to 6 weeks in patients with CRS for whom surgical management and multiple courses of oral antibiotics failed. Insufficient data are available to make a recommendation regarding the topical administration of antibiotics in patients with CRS.

## Nasal Irrigations

Most studies show nasal rinses with saline solution to be effective in alleviating symptoms and improving endoscopic appearance in patients with CRS.[87,88] Hypertonic saline has been shown to improve nasal mucociliary clearance compared with isotonic saline.[89] Side effects of saline irrigations, though uncommon, include nasal irritation, tearing, ear symptoms, cough, and headaches.[6]

## Leukotriene Modifiers

Leukotrienes are upregulated in nasal polyposis and asthma. Results are mixed regarding their role in the management of CRS. A study of 36 patients with CRS treated with a leukotriene modifier in addition to standard management showed a significant improvement in symptom scores for a wide variety of complaints, including headache, facial pain, ear discomfort, and purulent nasal discharge. Overall, 72% of patients noted improvement.[90] More rigorous studies are needed to evaluate the efficacy of leukotriene modifiers in treating CRS and its subtypes.

## Surgery

Each practitioner may have a unique algorithm for conservatively managing CRS, which typically includes nasal irrigations and a trial of topical corticosteroids, and may also involve therapies such as leukotriene modifiers, oral or topical antibiotic preparations, allergy management, or oral steroids. For symptoms refractory to a patient-specific medical treatment regimen, surgical intervention can be offered.

Several systematic reviews have analyzed the effectiveness of endoscopic sinus surgery. In a review that reported the subjective experience of 1713 patients who underwent endoscopic sinus surgery, 63% reported a "very good" result, which was defined as complete symptom resolution or fewer than two episodes of rhinosinusitis per year.[91] In this study, 12% of patients required revision surgery and 1.6% of patients experienced a surgical complication. The study did not, however, differentiate between CRS with and without nasal polyps. In general, the presence of polyps in patients with CRS has been shown to portend a less favorable result from surgery.[92]

A prospective study by Smith and colleagues evaluated the impact of endoscopic sinus surgery on quality of life and symptoms after failed medical treatment.[93] The authors concluded that significant evidence shows that endoscopic sinus surgery is effective in improving symptoms and quality of life in patients with CRS. Patients with CRS with and without nasal polyps were included in this meta-analysis. However, not all reviews have supported the role of functional endoscopic sinus surgery (FESS) in treating patients with CRS. A recent Cochrane review that included three randomized controlled studies concluded that FESS is not superior to medical treatment in patients with CRS.[94]

An observational study of 3128 prospectively enrolled patients undergoing sinus surgery in England and Wales showed significant improvement in symptom scores at 3, 12, and 36 months in patients with CRS, including those with nasal polyps.[95] In another prospective study, 160 patients with CRS with and without polyps were nonrandomly treated with wither medical therapy alone or surgery plus medical therapy. The medically managed group had less-severe sinus disease, as would be expected from a nonrandomized study. At 3 months, the surgically treated group showed more improvement than the nonsurgically treated group, but adjustments were not made for pretreatment disease severity.[96]

A recent randomized controlled trial included 109 patients with CRS with extensive polyps. Fifty-three patients received a tapering course of steroids for 2 weeks, whereas the remainder underwent endoscopic sinus surgery. All patients received nasal steroids for 1 year postoperatively. At 6 and 12 months, a significant improvement in symptom scores and polyp size was seen in both arms. The surgically treated group showed a significant advantage over the medically managed group for nasal obstruction, loss of smell at 6 months, and polyp size at 6 and 12 months.[97]

## Balloon Sinus Dilation

Balloon catheters have been used selectively as a new tool to achieve sinus ostial patency.[98] Since 2002, more than 20,000 patients have been treated worldwide with balloon sinus dilation.[99] Using traditional endoscopes for visualization, the balloon is passed into the natural sinus ostium and inflated to dilate the sinus outflow tract. The frontal, sphenoid, and maxillary sinuses can be managed in this fashion.[98]

After an initial feasibility study on cadavers showed successful dilation of the targeted sinus ostia without evidence of injury to adjacent structures,[100] a human pilot study was conducted in which all ostia were dilated without adverse events or direct mucosal injury. Although the frontal and sphenoid sinuses dilated with ease, some difficulty was reported in dilating the maxillary ostium in 5 of 10 patients.[101]

One study reported successful dilation of the osteomeatal complex in 55 of 58 patients via a transantral approach with endoscopic guidance. Statistically significant improvement in symptom scores was reported after 6 months, and 97% of the procedures were completed under local anesthesia with or without minimal intravenous sedation.[102] Another study showed long-term improvement in symptom scores and endoscopic patency rates after balloon sinus dilation, with no reported adverse events.[103]

The safety profile of balloon sinus dilation is supported in the literature. A retrospective review of 1036 patients who had 3276 sinuses treated documented two cerebrospinal fluid leaks and six cases of minor bleeding requiring cautery or packing. All eight events occurred in patients in whom balloon dilation was used in conjunction with conventional endoscopic sinus surgery. Analysis of an FDA database showed two reports of penetration of the lamina papyracea and one skull base defect in a "hybrid" case (traditional endoscopic surgery combined with balloon sinus dilation). Two cases of device malfunction were found, in which the balloon broke away from the catheter.[98]

One criticism of balloon dilation for CRS is that diseased bone that contributes to chronic sinus inflammation is not removed and may not be remodeled by the balloon as readily as healthy bone.[104,105]

Balloon dilation of sinus ostia may have a role in relieving obstruction and improving ventilation of sinuses in selected patients with CRS. The data are early but seem promising. Balloon technology is also currently being translated for office use. Further studies and long-term data are needed to define which patients will be best treated with this therapy.

## SUMMARY

CRS is a multifactorial inflammatory process involving the lining membrane of the nose and paranasal sinuses. Nasal obstruction, one of the principal symptoms of CRS, is a frequent presenting functional complaint in patients pursuing rhinoplasty. Despite the tendency to ascribe nasal obstruction to anatomic derangements such as nasal septal deviation, hypertrophic inferior turbinates, or narrow nasal valves, the rhinoplasty surgeon must have a systematic approach to patients with nasal obstruction to recognize and diagnose CRS. A focused history that elicits additional sinonasal complaints should direct the surgeon to obtain an endoscopic examination of the nasal cavity and middle meatus or imaging of the paranasal sinuses. Once CRS is diagnosed, medical therapy is typically the first line of treatment. In patients who remain symptomatic despite individualized medical management, endoscopic sinus surgery has been shown to provide symptomatic relief.

## REFERENCES

1. Pleis JR, Lethbridge-Cejku M. Summary of health statistics for U.S. adults: National Health Interview Survey. 2006. Vital Health Stat 10 2007;235: 1–153.
2. Gliklich RE, Metson R. Economic implications of chronic rhinosinusitis. Otolaryngol Head Neck Surg 1995;113:104–9.
3. Murphy MP, Fishman P, Short SO, et al. Health care utilization and cost among adults with chronic rhinosinusitis enrolled in a health maintenance organization. Otolaryngol Head Neck Surg 2002; 127:367–76.
4. Bhattacharyya N. Ambulatory sinus and nasal surgery in the United States: demographics and perioperative outcomes. Laryngoscope 2010;120: 635–8.
5. Rosenfeld RM, Andes D, Bhattacharyya N, et al. Clinical practice guideline: adult sinusitis. Otolaryngol Head Neck Surg 2007;137(Suppl 3):S1–31.
6. Fokkens WJ, Lund VJ, Mullol J, et al. European position paper on nasal polyps. Rhinology 2007; 45(Suppl 20):1–139.
7. Bachert C, Wagenmann M, Hauser U, et al. IL-5 synthesis is upregulated in human nasal polyp tissue. J Allergy Clin Immunol 1997;99(6 Pt 1): 837–42.
8. Hedman J, Kaprio J, Poussa T, et al. Prevalence of asthma, aspirin intolerance, nasal polyposis and chronic obstructive pulmonary disease in a population-based study. Int J Epidemiol 1999;28(4): 717–22.
9. Larsen K. The clinical relationship of nasal polyps to asthma. Allergy Asthma Proc 1996;17(5):243–9.
10. Settipane GA, Chafee FH. Nasal polyps in asthma and rhinitis. A review of 6,037 patients. J Allergy Clin Immunol 1977;59(1):17–21.

11. Caplin I, Haynes JT, Spahn J. Are nasal polyps an allergic phenomenon? Ann Allergy 1971;29(12):631–4.
12. Bent JP III, Kuhn FA. Diagnosis of allergic fungal sinusitis. Otolaryngol Head Neck Surg 1994;111(5):580–8.
13. Ferguson BJ. Eosinophilic mucin rhinosinusitis: a distinct clinicopathological entity. Laryngoscope 2000;110:799–813.
14. Slavin RG. Nasal polyps and sinusitis. JAMA 1997;278(22):1849–54.
15. Sturgess JM, Chao J, Wong J, et al. Cilia with defective radial spokes: a cause of human respiratory disease. N Engl J Med 1979;300(2):53–6.
16. Bhattacharyya N. The role of infection in chronic rhinosinusitis. Curr Allergy Asthma Rep 2002;2(6):500–6.
17. Zacharek MA, Krouse JH. The role of allergy in chronic rhinosinusitis. Curr Opin Otolaryngol Head Neck Surg 2003;11(3):196–200.
18. Jones NS. CT of the paranasal sinuses: a review of the correlation with clinical, surgical and histopathological findings. Clin Otolaryngol 2002;27(1):11–7.
19. Jones NS, Strobl A, Holland I. A study of the CT findings in 100 patients with rhinosinusitis and 100 controls. Clin Otolaryngol 1997;22(1):47–51.
20. Krause HF. Allergy and chronic rhinosinusitis. Otolaryngol Head Neck Surg 2003;128(1):14–6.
21. Stammberger H. Functional endoscopic sinus surgery. Philadelphia: B.C. Decker; 1991.
22. Lanza DC, Kennedy DW. Adult rhinosinusitis defined. Otolaryngol Head Neck Surg 1997;117(3 Pt 2):S1–7.
23. Benninger M. Rhinitis, sinusitis and their relationship to allergies. Am J Rhinol 1992;6:37–43.
24. Savolainen S. Allergy in patients with acute maxillary sinusitis. Allergy 1989;44(2):116–22.
25. Emanuel IA, Shah SB. Chronic rhinosinusitis: allergy and sinus computed tomography relationships. Otolaryngol Head Neck Surg 2000;123(6):687–91.
26. Grove R, Farrior J. Chronic hyperplastic sinusitis in allergic patients: a bacteriologic study of 200 operative cases. J Allergy Clin Immunol 1990;11:271–6.
27. Delaney JC. Aspirin idiosyncrasy in patients admitted for nasal polypectomy. Clin Otolaryngol 1976;1(1):27–30.
28. English G. Nasal polyposis. In: GM E, editor. Otolaryngology. Philadelphia: Harper and Row; 1985. p. 1–30.
29. Bachert C, Gevaert P, Holtappels G, et al. Total and specific IgE in nasal polyps is related to local eosinophilic inflammation. J Allergy Clin Immunol 2001;107(4):607–14.
30. Collins MM, Loughran S, Davidson P, et al. Nasal polyposis: prevalence of positive food and inhalant skin tests. Otolaryngol Head Neck Surg 2006;135(5):680–3.
31. Pang YT, Eskici O, Wilson JA. Nasal polyposis: role of subclinical delayed food hypersensitivity. Otolaryngol Head Neck Surg 2000;122(2):298–301.
32. Karlsson G, Holmberg K. Does allergic rhinitis predispose to sinusitis? Acta Otolaryngol Suppl 1994;515:26–8 [discussion: 9].
33. Lane AP, Pine HS, Pillsbury HC III. Allergy testing and immunotherapy in an academic otolaryngology practice: a 20- year review. Otolaryngol Head Neck Surg 2001;124(1):9–15.
34. Bousquet J, Van Cauwenberge P, Khaltaev N. Allergic rhinitis and its impact on asthma. J Allergy Clin Immunol 2001;108(Suppl 5):S147–334.
35. Slavin RG. Relationship of nasal disease and sinusitis to bronchial asthma. Ann Allergy 1982;49(2):76–9.
36. Nisioka GJ, Cook PR, Davis WE, et al. Functional endoscopic sinus surgery in patients with chronic sinusitis and asthma. Otolaryngol Head Neck Surg 1994;110(6):494–500.
37. Salvin RG, Cannon RE, Friedman WH, et al. Sinusitis and bronchial asthma. J Allergy Clin Immunol 1980;66(3):250–7.
38. Schwartz HJ, Thompson JS, Sher TH, et al. Occult sinus abnormalities in the asthmatic patient. Arch Intern Med 1987;147(12):2194–6.
39. Bresciani M, Paradis L, Des Roches A, et al. Rhinosinusitis in severe asthma. J Allergy Clin Immunol 2001;107(1):73–80.
40. Klossek JM, Neukirch F, Pribil C, et al. Prevalence of nasal polyposis in France: a cross- sectional, case-control study. Allergy 2005;60(2):233–7.
41. Collins MM, Pang YT, Loughran S, et al. Environmental risk factors and gender in nasal polyposis. Clin Otolaryngol 2002;27(5):314–7.
42. Zinreich SJ, Mattox DE, Kennedy DW, et al. Concha bullosa: CT evaluation. J Comput Assist Tomogr 1988;12:778–84.
43. Orlandi RR. A systematic analysis of septal deviation associated with rhinosinusitis. Laryngoscope 2010;120:1687–95.
44. Bolger WE, Butzin CA, Parsons DS. Paranasal sinus bony anatomic variations and mucosal abnormalities: CT analysis for endoscopic sinus surgery. Laryngoscope 1991;101(1 Pt 1):56–64.
45. Holbrook EH, Brown CL, Lyden ER, et al. Lack of significant correlation between rhinosinusitis symptoms and specific regions of sinus computer tomography scans. Am J Rhinol 2005;19(4):382–7.
46. Willner A, Choi SS, Vezina LG, et al. Intranasal anatomic variations in pediatric sinusitis. Am J Rhinol 1997;11(5):355–60.
47. Schubert MS. Allergic fungal sinusitis. Otolaryngol Clin North Am 2004;37(2):301–26.
48. Ponikau JU, Sherris DA, Kern EB, et al. The diagnosis and incidence of allergic fungal sinusitis. Mayo Clin Proc 1999;74(9):877–84.

49. Braun H, Buzina W, Freudenschuss K, et al. Eosinophilic fungal rhinosinusitis: a common disorder in Europe? Laryngoscope 2003;113(2):264–9.

50. Orlandi RR, Marple BF. Fungus and chronic rhinosinusitis: weighing the evidence. Otolaryngol Head Neck Surg 2010;143(5):611–3.

51. Ebbens FA, Scadding GK, Badia L, et al. Amphotericin B nasal lavages: not a solution for patients with chronic rhinosinusitis. J Allergy Clin Immunol 2006;118(5):1149–56.

52. Lee JT, Kennedy DW, Palmer JN, et al. The incidence of concurrent osteitis in patients with chronic rhinosinusitis: a clinicopathological study. Am J Rhinol 2006;20(3):278–82.

53. Kennedy DW, Senior BA, Gannon FH, et al. Histology and histomorphometry of ethmoid bone in chronic rhinosinusitis. Laryngoscope 1998;108 (4 Pt 1):502–7.

54. Perloff JR, Gannon FH, Bolger WE, et al. Bone involvement in sinusitis: an apparent pathway for the spread of disease. Laryngoscope 2000;110(12): 2095–9.

55. Bezerra T, Padua F, Gebrim E, et al. Biofilms in chronic rhinosinusitis. Otolaryngol Head Neck Surg 2011;144(4):612–6.

56. Costerton W, Veeh R, Shirtliff M, et al. The application of biofilm science to the study and control of chronic bacterial infections. J Clin Invest 2003; 112:1466–77.

57. Post JC. Direct evidence of bacterial biofilms in otitis media. Laryngoscope 2001;111:2083–94.

58. Post JC, Stoodley P, Hall-Stoodley, et al. The role of biofilms in otolaryngologic infections. Curr Opin Otolaryngol Head Neck Surg 2004;12:185–90.

59. Zuliani G, Carron M, Gurrola J, et al. Identification of adenoid biofilms in chronic rhinosinusitis. Int J Pediatr Otorhinolaryngol 2006;70:1613–7.

60. Perloff JR, Palmer JN. Evidence of bacterial biofilms on frontal recess stents in patients with chronic rhinosinusitis. Am J Rhinol 2004;18:377–80.

61. Cryer J, Schipor I, Perloff JR, et al. Evidence of bacterial biofilms in human chronic rhinosinusitis. ORL J Otorhinolaryngol Relat Spec 2004;66:155–8.

62. Ferguson BJ, Stolz DB. Demonstration of biofilm in human bacterial chronic rhinosinusitis. Am J Rhinol 2005;19:452–7.

63. Bernstein JM, Ballow M, Schlievert PM, et al. A superantigen hypothesis for the pathogenesis of chronic hyperplastic sinusitis with massive nasal polyposis. Am J Rhinol 2003;17:321–6.

64. Al-Rawi MM, Edelstein DR, Erlandson RA. Changes in nasal epithelium in patients with severe chronic sinusitis: a clinicopathologic and electron microscopic study. Laryngoscope 1998;108(12):1816–23.

65. Chen Y, Dales R, Lin M. The epidemiology of chronic rhinosinusitis in Canadians. Laryngoscope 2003;113(7):1199–205.

66. Greisner WA III, Settipane GA. Hereditary factor for nasal polyps. Allergy Asthma Proc 1996;17(5): 283–6.

67. Morinaka S, Ichimiya M, Nakamura H. Detection of Helicobacter pylori in nasal and maxillary sinus specimens from patients with chronic sinusitis. Laryngoscope 2003;113(9):1557–63.

68. Ozdek A, Cirak MY, Samim E, et al. A possible role of Helicobacter pylori in chronic rhinosinusitis: a preliminary report. Laryngoscope 2003;113(4): 679–82.

69. DelGaudio JM. Direct nasopharyngeal reflux of gastric acid is a contributing factor in refractory chronic rhinosinusitis. Laryngoscope 2005;115(6): 946–57.

70. Gutman M, Houser S. Iatrogenic maxillary sinus recirculation and beyond. Ear Nose Throat J 2003; 82(1):61–3.

71. Vento SI, Ertama LO, Hytonen ML, et al. Nasal polyposis: clinical course during 20 years. Ann Allergy Asthma Immunol 2000;85(3): 209–14.

72. Lund VJ, Kennedy DW. Quantification for staging sinusitis. The Staging and Therapy Group. Ann Otol Rhinol Laryngol Suppl 1995;167:17–21.

73. Lavigne F, Cameron L, Renzi PM, et al. Intrasinus administration of topical budesonide to allergic patients with chronic rhinosinusitis following surgery. Laryngoscope 2002;112(5):858–64.

74. Lund VJ, Black JH, Szabo LZ, et al. Efficacy and tolerability of budesonide aqueous nasal spray in chronic rhinosinusitis patients. Rhinology 2004; 42(2):57–62.

75. Deuschl H, Drettner B. Nasal polyps treated by beclomethasone nasal aerosol. Rhinology 1977;15(1): 17–23.

76. Small CB, Hernandez J, Reyes A, et al. Efficacy and safety of mometasone furoate nasal spray in nasal polyposis. J Allergy Clin Immunol 2005; 116(6):1275–81.

77. Stjarne P, Mosges R, Jorissen M, et al. A randomized controlled trial of mometasone furoate nasal spray for the treatment of nasal polyposis. Arch Otolaryngol Head Neck Surg 2006;132(2):179–85.

78. Stjarne P, Blomgren K, Caye-Thomasen P, et al. The efficacy and safety of once-daily mometasone furoate nasal spray in nasal polyposis: a randomized, double-blind, placebo-controlled study. Acta Otolaryngol 2006;126(6): 606–12.

79. Holm AF, Fokkens WJ, Godthelp T, et al. A 1-year placebo-controlled study of intranasal fluticasone propionate aqueous nasal spray in patients with perennial allergic rhinitis: a safety and biopsy study. Clin Otolaryngol 1998;23(1):69–73.

80. Bielory L, Blaiss M, Fineman SM, et al. Concerns about intranasal corticosteroids for over-the-counter

use: position statement of the Joint Task Force for the American Academy of Allergy, Asthma and Immunology and the American College of Allergy, Asthma and Immunology. Ann Allergy Asthma Immunol 2006; 96(4):514–25.

81. Benitez P, Alobid I, De Haro J, et al. A short course of oral prednisone followed by intranasal budesonide is an effective treatment of severe nasal polyps. Laryngoscope 2006;116(5):770–5.

82. Hissaria P, Smith W, Wormald PJ, et al. Short course of systemic corticosteroids in sinonasal polyposis: a double-blind, randomized, placebo-controlled trial with evaluation of outcome measures. J Allergy Clin Immunol 2006;118(1): 128–33.

83. Cave A, Arlett P, Lee E. Inhaled and nasal corticosteroids: factors affecting the risks of systemic adverse effects. Pharmacol Ther 1999;83(3): 153–79.

84. Hashiba M, Baba S. Efficacy of long-term administration of clarithromycin in the treatment of intractable chronic sinusitis. Acta Otolaryngol Suppl 1996;525:73–8.

85. Desrosiers MY, Salas-Prato M. Treatment of chronic rhinosinusitis refractory to other treatments with topical antibiotic therapy delivered by means of a large-particle nebulizer: results of a controlled trial. Otolaryngol Head Neck Surg 2001;125(3): 265–9.

86. Scheinberg PA, Otsuji A. Nebulized antibiotics for the treatment of acute exacerbations of chronic rhinosinusitis. Ear Nose Throat J 2002;81(9):648–52.

87. Bachmann G, Hommel G, Michel O. Effect of irrigation of the nose with isotonic salt solution on adult patients with chronic paranasal sinus disease. Eur Arch Otorhinolaryngol 2000;257(10):537–41.

88. Taccariello M, Parikh A, Darby Y, et al. Nasal douching as a valuable adjunct in the management of chronic rhinosinusitis. Rhinology 1999;37(1): 29–32.

89. Talbot AR, Herr TM, Parsons DS. Mucociliary clearance and buffered hypertonic saline solution. Laryngoscope 1997;107(4):500–3.

90. Parnes SM, Chuma AV. Acute effects of antileukotrienes on sinonasal polyposis and sinusitis. Ear Nose Throat J 2000;79(1):18–20, 4–5.

91. Terris MH, Davidson TM. Review of published results for endoscopic sinus surgery. Ear Nose Throat J 1994;73(8):574–80.

92. Deal RT, Kountakis SE. Significance of nasal polyps in chronic rhinosinusitis: symptoms and surgical outcomes. Laryngoscope 2004;114(11 I):1932–5.

93. Smith TL, Mendolia-Loffredo S, Loehrl TA, et al. Predictive factors and outcomes in endoscopic sinus surgery for chronic rhinosinusitis. Laryngoscope 2005;115(12):2199.

94. Khalil HS, Nunez DA. Functional endoscopic sinus surgery for chronic rhinosinusitis. Cochrane Database Syst Rev 2006;3:CD004458.

95. Hopkins C, Browne JP, Slack R, et al. Complications of surgery for nasal polyposis and chronic rhinosinusitis: the results of a national audit in England and Wales. Laryngoscope 2006;116(8): 1494–9.

96. Gliklich RE, Metson R. Effect of sinus surgery on quality of life. Otolaryngol Head Neck Surg 1997; 117(1):12–7.

97. Alobid I, Benitez P, Bernal-Sprekelsen M, et al. Nasal polyposis and its impact on quality of life: comparison between the effects of medical and surgical treatments. Allergy 2005;60(4):452–8.

98. Kim E, Cutler JL. Balloon dilatation of the paranasal sinuses: a tool in sinus surgery. Otolaryngol Clin North Am 2009;42:847–56.

99. Slow JK, Kadah BA, Werner AJ. Balloon sinuplasty: a current hot topic in rhinology. Eur Arch Otorhinolaryngol 2008;265:509–11.

100. Bolger WE, Vaughan W. Catheter based dilation of the sinus ostia: initial safety and feasibility in a cadaver model. Am J Rhinol 2006;20(6):290–4.

101. Brown C, Bolger WE. Safety and feasibility of balloon catheter dilation of sinus ostia: a preliminary investigation. Ann Otol Rhinol Laryngol 2006; 115(4):293–9.

102. Stankiewicz J, Tami T, Truitt T, et al. Transantral endoscopically guided balloon dilation of the osteomeatal complex for chronic rhinosinusitis under local anesthesia. Am J Rhinol Allergy 2009;23:1–7.

103. Weiss RL, Church CA, Kuhn FA, et al. Long-term analysis of balloon catheter sinusotomy: two-year follow-up. Otolaryngol Head Neck Surg 2008;138: S38–46.

104. Melroy CT. The balloon dilating catheter as an instrument in sinus surgery. Otolaryngol Head Neck Surg 2008;139:S23–6.

105. Lanza DC, Kennedy DW. Balloon sinuplasty: not ready for prime time [commentary]. Ann Otol Rhinol Laryngol 2006;115(10):789–90.

# Allergic Rhinitis

James W. Mims, MD

## KEYWORDS

- Allergic rhinitis • Epidemiology • Diagnosis
- Immunotherapy • Environmental control

---

**Key Points**

- Physicians evaluating patients for functional nasal problems should be familiar with the diagnosis and treatment of allergic rhinitis.
- Allergic rhinitis is a common disorder that causes symptoms of rhinorrhea, sneezing, nasal itching, and nasal congestion.
- Allergic rhinitis also affects quality of life, sleep, school performance, and productivity.
- Management options for allergic rhinitis include pharmacotherapy, environmental control, and immunotherapy.
- Turbinate reduction may be useful in selected patients with allergic rhinitis.
- Nasal congestion secondary to allergic reaction has the potential to negatively affect the functional outcome of nasal esthetic procedures that narrow the nasal valve.

---

Facial plastic surgeons need to be familiar with common inflammatory conditions of the nose, as these affect nasal function. Frequently, nasal obstruction has both structural and inflammatory contributions and recognition of both is important. Counseling patients about coexisting nasal inflammation helps establish more realistic expectations of nasal surgical results and can be used to guide patients toward other effective treatments. One of the most common sources of nasal inflammation is allergic rhinitis. Although not life threatening, allergic rhinitis has a substantial affect on a patient's quality of life, sleep, school performance, and productivity.[1] Physicians should also be aware of the association of allergic rhinitis with other conditions, such as asthma. Asthma is both underdiagnosed and suboptimally controlled in the United States.[2] This article focuses on the epidemiology, diagnosis, and treatment of allergic rhinitis. As there are articles elsewhere in this issue on the related topics of nonallergic rhinitis, allergic

pharmacotherapy, and the united airway, these topics will not be covered in detail.

## DEFINITION AND GENETICS OF ALLERGIC RHINITIS

Allergic rhinitis is clinically defined in the 2008 Allergic Rhinitis and its Impact on Asthma (ARIA) Guidelines as "a symptomatic disorder of the nose induced after allergen exposure by an IgE-mediated inflammation."[3] Allergic patients have a genetic tendency to produce an inflammatory response to particles that are normally harmless. It is the inflammation that causes their symptoms. As the inflammation is unnecessary for nonpathogenic particles (such as pollen), these are described as hypersensitivity reactions. Atopy is the genetic predisposition to develop allergic hypersensitivity reactions. Atopic disease generally causes local inflammation at the surface of exposure and is classified as such. Examples

Financial disclosures: None.
Department of Otolaryngology, Wake Forest School of Medicine, Medical Center Boulevard, Winston-Salem, NC 27157, USA
E-mail address: wmims@wfubmc.edu

are allergic conjunctivitis, allergic rhinitis, allergic asthma, atopic dermatitis, and food allergies. Atopic individuals with one allergic condition tend to be at risk for others.

The underlying genetics of allergic individuals is not well understood but appears to be complex. Initially, it was speculated that the genetics of allergy were based in alterations of the inflammatory process. Studies that looked for particular changes in the genetic code (single nucleotide polymorphisms or SNIPs) targeted the components of allergic inflammation. Allergic individuals were found to have more SNIPs in genes coding for many components of allergic inflammation, including interleukin (IL)-4, IL-13, and T-cell receptors, than nonallergic controls.[4] More than 100 SNIPs have been identified as more prevalent in allergic populations than in controls; but, individual SNIP studies often have poor reproducibility.[4] Larger studies that were hypothesis independent (such as Genome Wide Association [GWA] studies) compared thousands of known human SNIPs in allergic versus nonallergic populations. GWA studies have been mostly performed in allergic asthma. These studies identified different gene candidates that tended not to be linked directly to the allergic inflammatory cascade.[5] It is likely that a combination of factors of innate immunity and variable changes in the regulation of inflammation may both contribute toward allergic hypersensitivity. Genetically, allergic rhinitis is a heterogenic disease.[5]

This is perhaps best illustrated in atopic dermatitis. A defect in the protein fillagrin has been identified in about one-third of individuals with atopic dermatitis.[6] Fillagrin is a protein that helps connect or seal the outer layer of keratinocytes, and it is speculated that the genetic "loss of function" make the skin barrier more porous. One could speculate that allergic disease may require a combination of several different factors in a single individual, explaining the heterogeneity of disease. An individual with faulty innate immunity (a barrier defect like fillagrin) combined with a genetic tendency promoting inflammation may manifest allergic disease. Additionally, allergic individuals must also recognize allergen epitopes with preformed HLA, T-cell, and B-cell receptors, which may contribute to why different allergies develop.

The importance of the variety of genetic findings is that patients with similar allergic phenotypes (such as allergic rhinitis to grass pollen) may have different underlying genetics. In allergy, studies tend to differ by ethnicity and region and commonly contradict each other. Also, allergic and nonallergic rhinitis likely occur across a continuum rather than being distinctly separate processes.

# BASIC IMMUNOLOGY OF ALLERGY

Although there are 6 types of Gel and Coombs hypersensitivity reactions, the Gel and Coombs Type I reaction (immunoglobulin E [IgE]-mediated hypersensitivity) is classically seen in allergic disease. During sensitization, an allergen is recognized by an antigen-presenting cell (APC) and presented to a T-helper cell lymphocyte. The allergic patient is required to have specific HLA receptors on the APC and a specific T-cell receptor for this communication to take place. T-helper cells that are biased toward promoting allergic inflammation are called TH2 cells.[7] TH2 cells present the allergen (or allergic epitope) to a B lymphocyte, which must also have a B-cell receptor for that specific allergen. In the presence of allergic cytokines (such as IL-4) the B cell can change into an IgE-producing plasma cell for that particular allergen. The IgE produced travels through the circulation and tissue to bind to IgE receptors on mast cells and basophils.

If a patient is reexposed to the allergen and has allergen-specific IgE (sIgE) antibodies bound to their mast cells, it may cause the mast cell or basophil to degranulate, releasing inflammatory mediators, such as histamine. Histamine binds to histamine receptors on endothelial cells and vascular smooth muscle causing vasodilation and increased permeability.[8] The patient experiences rhinorrhea and nasal congestion. Other mediators promote more inflammation such as IL-5, which promotes eosinophilia, and leukotrienes, which recruit more inflammatory cells. The promotion of more inflammation is balanced by factors that down-regulate inflammations, such as IL-10. Down-regulation appears to be partially controlled by specialized T lymphoctyes (T-regs).[9]

# EPIDEMIOLOGY OF ALLERGIC RHINITIS

Allergic rhinitis is a common condition in the United States and the world and is increasing in developed countries.[10] Four relevant concepts to know about the epidemiology of allergic rhinitis are:

1. Prevalence
2. Cost
3. The "allergic march"
4. The "hygiene hypothesis".

In the United States, the 2009 National Health Interview Survey conducted by the Centers for Disease Control and Prevention reported that 17.7 million adults or 7.8% of those surveyed had been diagnosed with "hay fever" in the preceding 12 months[11]; 7.2 million children were reported to have "hay fever" and 8.2 million

(11%) were reported to have "respiratory allergy" in the preceding 12 months.[12] There is a difference between a survey for respiratory allergies and having a history and positive allergy test, however. In Sweden, by questionnaire alone, 14.2% were allergic as compared with 9.1% who were positive by questionnaire and skin test.[3]

The direct cost of allergic rhinitis includes medication and physician visits. In 2011, Meltzer and Bukstein[13] estimated the direct medical cost of allergic rhinitis at $3.4 billion in the United States. Indirect costs of missed work and lost productivity are more difficult to quantify. Given the quality of life impairment, the indirect costs are also likely to be substantial.

Because allergic rhinitis occurs as a result of genetic predisposition and environmental exposure, there is an accumulation of evidence to support the allergic or atopic "march." This is the concept that atopic individuals often have eczema and food allergies in infancy followed by allergic rhinitis and asthma, which peaks in teenagers and young adults.[14] The specifics of the allergic march seem to vary substantially in different cohorts, however.

A final important epidemiologic concept is the "hygiene hypothesis."[15] This is the controversial theory that infections early in life are protective against the later development of atopic disease. The theory is that T cells are more biased toward allergic inflammation at birth and early infections change their bias toward a nonallergic inflammatory pattern (TH1 cytokine profile) more appropriate for viral and bacterial infections. There are large well-done studies that both support and refute this theory.[15,16]

## DIAGNOSIS OF ALLERGIC RHINITIS
### History

A patient's symptom history is the most important element in determining allergic rhinitis. Allergy tests are frequently positive in individuals without significant clinical manifestations, and allergy tests do not make the diagnosis in isolation. Unfortunately, many of the symptoms in allergic rhinitis are also present in nonallergic rhinitis and chronic rhinosinusitis. The primary symptoms of allergic rhinitis are sneezing, nasal obstruction, rhinorrhea, and nasal itching.[3] Anterior rhinorrhea may be a more specific sign of allergic rhinitis than postnasal drip alone.[17]

Allergy should be suspected if symptoms are provoked by exposure to known allergens. If symptoms are exacerbated during a certain time of the year, such as when pollen counts are elevated, this would suggest allergy, although the

positive predictive values of specific patient-reported exposures are disappointing.[18] Patients allergic to dander may also provide a history of symptoms when exposed in a home or building where the animal resides. Other allergic patients have symptoms most of the year. Most patients with allergic rhinitis are polysensitized, which complicates pairing their history with patterns of exposure.[3]

Allergic rhinitis is frequently divided by whether the symptoms are present intermittently or persistently. Classically, allergic rhinitis is divided into seasonal allergic rhinitis (SAR) or perennial allergic rhinitis (PAR); however, the ARIA guidelines recommend intermittent allergic rhinitis (IAR) and persistent allergic rhinitis, as they concluded that there were too many exceptions to the seasonal model, especially with dust mites and molds.[3] Persistent allergic rhinitis is defined as more than 4 consecutive days per week or more than 4 consecutive weeks.[19] IAR tends to have symptoms of sneezing, itching, and rhinorrhea, whereas PAR's hallmark is nasal obstruction.

Severity of symptoms varies in allergic rhinitis and is subjective. The ARIA guidelines classify allergic rhinitis as moderate or severe when sleep disturbance or impairment of daily activities, work, or school is present (Table 1).[3]

Coexisting symptoms of wheezing or conjunctival irritation may help differentiate allergic rhinitis from nonallergic disease, as well as affect evaluation and treatment decisions. The patient's history of other atopic disorders, such as childhood food

| Table 1 ARIA classification of allergic rhinitis | |
|---|---|
| Intermittent | Symptoms are present <4 days a week or <4 consecutive weeks |
| Persistent | Symptoms are present >4 days per week and more than 4 consecutive weeks |
| Mild | None of the "Moderate/Severe" criteria present |
| Moderate/Severe | One or more of the following are present: Sleep disturbance Impairment of daily activities, leisure, and/or sport Impairment of school or work Troublesome symptoms |

Adapted from Bousquet J, Khaltaev N, Cruz AA, et al. Allergic Rhinitis and its Impact on Asthma (ARIA) 2008 update (in collaboration with the World Health Organization, GA(2)LEN and AllerGen). Allergy 2008;63(Suppl 86):8–160.

allergy or atopic dermatitis, may also support the diagnosis of allergic rhinitis.

A family history of allergies may also be useful, but allergic rhinitis does not follow simple Mendelian inheritance. Twin studies have found the proband concordance of asthma in monozygotic twins to be only 0.28 to 0.63.[20] In a large cohort in Sweden, family history of allergy had an odds ratio of 1.3 in predicting a positive skin-prick test in the child.[10]

### Physical Findings in Allergic Rhinitis

Anterior rhinoscopy may be useful in considering allergic rhinitis, but physical findings are nonspecific and may be present intermittently.[21] Inferior turbinates are generally enlarged and described as pale or boggy, but the specificity of these observations has not been carefully examined. Mucus may be more abundant or seen stranding between the turbinate and septum. Polyps are also a sign of chronic nasal inflammation, but curiously are not seen more frequently in allergic patients.[22]

During acute attacks, allergy sufferers have been observed to wrinkle their face and wipe their nose, especially children. A supranasal tip crease may develop from frequently lifting the nasal tip.[23] Fine wrinkles on the lower eyelid are frequently present. Other visual findings include venous congestion and swelling of the lower lids, which give the patient the appearance of being chronically tired. The conjunctiva may have prominent vessels or thickening of the scleral surface of the eyelids. Increased mucus secretion from the eye may be present.[23] Some have observed longer eyelashes in allergic patients, which may help protect the eye from allergens.

Oral pharyngeal findings may include mucus, which tends to drain on the sides. Erythema and edema of the posterior pharyngeal wall may be observed and this is also sometimes greatest on the lateral edges.

Inhaled allergen challenges have produced laryngeal edema and stranding mucus.[24] Auscultation for wheezing is also recommended if the patient is suspected of being allergic.

### Testing for Allergic Rhinitis

The diagnosis of allergy is primarily a clinical diagnosis, as positive allergy tests are frequently seen in individuals without allergic clinical symptoms. Furthermore, allergic and nonallergic rhinitis symptoms overlap substantially. In individuals with clinical symptoms and correlating positive allergy tests, however, improvement has been demonstrated with allergy medication, environmental control, and allergic desensitization (also known as allergen immunotherapy). Allergy testing is imperfect, but useful.

In a 2009 survey sponsored by the Centers for Disease Control and Prevention, 11.8% self-reported "respiratory allergies"[12]; however, more than 4 times that number have a positive skin test. The Third National Health and Nutrition Survey examined the prevalence of positive skin-prick test (SPT) for a screen of inhalant allergens. It found that 53.9% of the 10,508 who were randomly tested had at least one positive SPT.[25] This disparity between clinical symptoms and skin testing is also displayed in a Swiss study. In the 1998 Swiss Study of Air Pollution and Lung Diseases (SAPALDIA), clinical allergic rhinitis was determined by surveying and testing 8329 randomly selected adults. They were asked, "In the past 12 months, did you suffer from allergic rhinitis, including hay fever?" or "Did you experience a runny or stuffy nose, the urge to sneeze, or itchy or watery eyes related to common allergen exposure?" The positive predictive power of an SPT predicting clinical allergic rhinitis in this study was 48.7%.[26] The following sections discuss the different types of allergy testing, but it is important to recognize that there is a significant amount of clinical judgment in deciding whom to test. The previously mentioned studies suggest that allergy testing should not be used as a screening test independent of clinical symptoms, as there is a significant false positive rate.

Allergy testing is helpful in determining to what patients might be allergic. There are different methods of allergy testing that are subdivided into challenge tests, skin tests, and IgE measurement.

### Challenge Testing

Challenge testing is the exposure of an individual to an allergen and observing for an allergic reaction. Some of the first studies of allergic disease used conjunctival challenges with pollen.[27] For allergic rhinitis, it would involve placing allergen in the nose or placing the subject in a room with circulating allergen (an environmental exposure chamber). Challenge testing is used as the "gold standard" in food allergy[28] but is less agreed on in inhalant allergy testing. It might seem intuitive that challenge testing would be the gold standard for allergic rhinitis. If one placed ragweed pollen in the nose and the individual developed rhinorrhea and sniffling, then the person would be allergic to ragweed; however, challenge testing for inhalant allergens tends to exceed amounts encountered in natural exposures. Also, a single challenge may elicit a different response than a seasonal exposure. Perhaps for these reasons, challenge testing has not correlated optimally with clinical symptoms.[3] Additionally, challenge testing is difficult to standardize and suffers from subjective responses.[29] As such, challenge testing is relegated to research for allergic rhinitis.

## Skin Testing

Skin testing is the most widely used testing for allergies in the United States. An extract of an inhaled allergen is placed beneath the skin's surface via scratch, prick, or intradermal injection. If mast cells in the skin degranulate after allergen exposure, histamine and other mediators produce a wheal (local edema) and flare (erythema). The skin reaction is compared with positive (histamine) and negative (diluent) controls and graded (or read) by the tester. Skin-testing results may vary by technique, area of the body, test interpreter, medications, and allergen extract, but serve as a useful and effective tool for assessing the risk of allergy.[30] A small risk of triggering a systemic allergic reaction is incurred with all types of skin testing.[21]

Scratch testing is not currently recommended, as reproducible results are difficult to obtain.[3] Prick testing uses single-prick or multiprick devices to place the extract in the epidermis. Prick tests can be reproduced with practice and are favored for their safety, cost, and reasonable correlation to clinical disease. Intradermal tests use a needle to raise a small wheal and observe the wheal for growth and erythema. Single intradermal tests use more extract than prick tests alone and may generate a response when the prick test is negative. Studies have questioned if intradermal tests add any clinical value when the prick test is negative.[31] Intradermal tests using different dilutions of extract will show increasingly large wheals and flares in a sensitive subject.[30] Intradermal dilutional testing is used for antigen standardization and venom allergy testing, and was once widespread among otolaryngologists. As there is no agreed on gold standard for inhalant allergy testing, there is controversy about the best way to test for allergy. The most controversy surrounds using relatively high amounts of allergen applied intradermally.

## sIgE Testing

IgE is the molecule produced by plasma cells that recognizes the allergen and serves as the allergen receptor that triggers degranulation of mast cells and basophils. The plasma cells of the allergic individual constantly produce cloned specific IgE (sIgE) that is both bound on cells that express IgE receptors and free in the circulation. Free sIgE can be sampled in plasma or sera and is measured by allowing it to bind to an allergen (such as ragweed pollen) adhered to a matrix. The patient's bound IgE is tagged with a labeled anti-human IgE, which is then measured. This technique also allows the amount of sIgE to be indirectly quantified. In theory, any person with an IgE-mediated allergy would necessarily produce sIgE to that allergen; however, technical issues exist.[32]

sIgE testing has undergone several evolutions of technology and is currently judged to be slightly less sensitive than skin-prick testing. Advantages include that multiple tests can be run off a single blood draw, results are not suppressed with antihistamine use, and interpretation is not subjective.

Higher sIgE levels correlate with stronger skin-test reactions, and lower sIgE levels correlate with weaker skin reactions. Some evidence suggests that the higher the sIgE level, the more likely it is that the allergy is clinically present. A clear example of this relationship is in food allergy testing. In IgE mediated food allergy, sIgE levels correlate with the probability that the blinded food challenge will be positive.[33] Surprisingly, the degree of skin reactivity and level of sIgE have not correlated well with the severity of clinical symptoms.[34] The concept that strongly positive test results predict a higher probability of clinical allergy but not greater symptom severity is somewhat counterintuitive.

## Total IgE Testing

Total IgE can also be measured and again it is intuitive that allergic individuals would have high levels of total IgE. However, total IgE has not been found to be as helpful as sIgE in determining who is allergic and who is not. This is partly because other inflammatory conditions, such as asthma, chronic eosinophilic sinusitis, and smoking, are associated with high total IgE. Also, many patients with allergic rhinitis defined by positive tests and history have total IgE in the normal range.[32,35]

## Testing Summary

Allergic rhinitis is a clinical diagnosis, not a test result. Testing is useful in separating allergic rhinitis and nonallergic rhinitis but loses specificity when applied independent of clinical impression. The accuracy of allergy testing also varies among different allergens. For some allergens, the extracts used in testing are standardized and the specific protein epitopes that bind to the IgE are shared among most allergic individuals. Cat and ragweed are examples of standardized extracts with a prominent "major allergens"; however, other allergens, especially molds, are not standardized and have multiple allergenic epitopes but no "major allergen." Most allergenic sources have multiple allergens and a "major allergen" is determined when more than 50% of the sensitized population reacts to that particular allergen.

## TREATMENT OF ALLERGIC RHINITIS

Treatment of allergic rhinitis is traditionally divided into 3 categories: pharmacotherapy, environmental control, and immunotherapy (or desensitization). Because this article targets surgeons, we also discuss the role of surgical interventions. As pharmacotherapy is covered in depth in the article "Pharmacotherapy" by Chaaban and Corey elsewhere in this issue, the discussion in this article is cursory.

### Pharmacotherapy

Pharmacologic management of allergic rhinitis is used in most patients, and billions of dollars are spent in allergic prescription and over-the-counter medications each year.[1] A brief comment on selecting the different categories of allergy medications is summarized in the following paragraphs.

Systemic steroids are highly effective at decreasing the inflammation from allergic rhinitis but carry a risk and side-effect profile that is difficult to justify when other options are available. For severe intermittent allergic rhinitis that is otherwise not well controlled, however, a short course may be reasonable.

Intranasal corticosteroids (INCSs), aside from systemic steroids, are the single most effective class of medical therapy for allergic rhinitis. There is little difference in clinical efficacy between available INCSs; however, differences in price, taste, and systemic effects exist. Local irritation, especially ulceration and bleeding from the nasal septum, is a common side effect with persistent use. Educating patients to spray parallel to the turbinates and to not angle the bottle toward the septum seems helpful in reducing local irritation in the author's experience. Although intermittent use has demonstrated efficacy, maximal efficacy of symptom control occurs after 7 to 10 days of use. As such, INCSs are perhaps not the best choice for intermittent use or as a rescue medication.[1]

Antihistamines are divided into first and second generations, with sedation being much less in the second-generation medications. Sedation with first-generation antihistamines can last into the following day and impairs work productivity, school performance, and driving. First-generation antihistamines do not have a rational role in the management of allergic rhinitis for most patients. Antihistamines help with rhinorrhea, itching, and sneezing, but are similar to placebo for nasal congestion. Antihistamines are often paired with decongestants for this reason. Antihistamines are receptor blockers and are probably more effective if taken before a known allergen exposure, but they also work relatively quickly and are practical as a rescue medication. Cetirizine,[36] fexofenadine,[37] and levocetirizine[38] provide greater symptom control than loratidine dosed at 10 mg in environmental exposure unit studies. Intranasal antihistamines also work well and have an additive affect when used with INCSa; however, taste and sedation are issues for some patients.[39]

Leukotriene modifiers are effective for allergic rhinitis, control symptoms comparable with loratidine, and have an added effect when combined with antihistamines, approaching INCSs.[40] Generally, leukotriene modifiers are used more in patients with allergic rhinitis and asthma.

Cromolyn requires frequent dosing and has mild efficacy, but has excellent safety.[1]

Decongestants are effective with nasal congestion and rhinorrhea but can have significant side effects, including sleep disruption and hypertension. They are best fitted for intermittent allergic rhinitis or as a rescue medication in young adults without hypertension.[1]

### Environmental Control

Environmental avoidance is recommended in multiple position papers, but has poor support from controlled studies in consistently improving symptoms. It is helpful to classify the studies into 3 groups.

#### Allergic subjects are physically removed from allergenic source

Mostly looking at allergic asthma, studies have shown that moving sensitized patients to an allergen-free location improves symptoms. In one study, schoolchildren with asthma and allergic to dust mites were enrolled in a school located at a high altitude in the Alps where dust mites could not survive. They had significant improvement in their asthma.[41] Similar improvements in asthma are sometimes seen when patients are admitted into a hospital. Although effective, this strategy is frequently impractical.

#### Environmental control techniques with allergen measurement as the outcome

Multiple studies will measure the amount of allergen in the air or grams of dust and then apply an intervention, such as dust-mite covers.

Postintervention measurements are compared for statistical significance. By this standard, many interventions, including dust-mite covers,[42] acaracides,[43,44] vacuum cleaning,[45] HEPA filters,[46] washing linens,[47] removing carpets,[48] and washing pets[49] are effective. Of note, washing cats reduces levels for only a single day. Despite reduction of measured allergens, the clinical implication of this is less certain.

### Environmental control techniques with allergy symptom outcomes

Improvement of symptoms or decreased medication use is much more difficult to demonstrate. An example of this type of study would be a randomized blinded placebo-controlled trial published in the *New England Journal of Medicine* that looked at the effect of dust-mite covers on allergic rhinitis in 232 dust mite–sensitized patients. The investigators showed no difference in their clinical outcome measures.[50] In many cases, the reduction of allergen seems to be insufficient to benefit the allergic patients. One of the interesting features of allergic reactions is how a small exposure can trigger symptoms. Studies that have used rigorous environmental control with multiple interventions have shown some success.[51]

In allergic rhinitis, patients wishing to use environmental controls as a strategy should commit to multimodalities and stringent interventions (removing carpets or pets), or expect modest results.[51] When paired with medical therapy, environmental controls and avoidance can result in subjective improvement in some patients. This topic is also discussed elsewhere in this issue.

### Surgery as an Adjunct for Allergic Rhinitis?

Nasal congestion is a primary symptom of allergic rhinitis and is likely the symptom most responsible for the impairment of quality of life and sleep in those with allergic rhinitis.[1] Hypertrophy of the inferior turbinate is partially responsible for the nasal obstruction. A recent study randomized 55 patients with allergic rhinitis to radiofrequency reduction of the inferior turbinates or intranasal mometasone spray. At 1 year, turbinate reduction provided significantly better decreased nasal resistance, significantly improved congestion subjectively assessed by visual analog scale, and similar improvements in a validated quality-of-life instrument as compared with intranasal mometasone. The turbinate reduction group was significantly better in the domains of sleep and nasal symptoms.[52] Two other studies support these findings. Mori and colleagues[53] reported benefit in quality of life in patients with perennial allergic rhinitis 5 years after submucosal reduction of the turbinates. Lin and colleagues[54] reported improved symptoms in 108 subjects with allergic rhinitis refractory to medical therapy after radiofrequency turbinate reduction assessed 1 year after surgery. Take together, these 3 studies provide data that support considering turbinate reduction for allergic rhinitis in selected patients. Surgery may also have a role when allergic rhinitis coexists with nasal valve collapse, deviated septum, nasal polyps, adenoid hypertrophy, or chronic sinusitis, in the author's opinion.

### Immunotherapy

Although pharmacotherapy, environmental avoidance, and possibly surgery may help manage allergic rhinitis, only immunotherapy has the potential to permanently decrease or resolve the underlying allergic inflammation. Allergen immunotherapy is the regular exposure of the sensitized patient to the allergen(s) to which the patients is sensitized so as to promote tolerance.[55] Inhalant allergen immunotherapy is classified by the route the allergen extract is delivered. Immunotherapy can be provided subcutaneously (shots), sublingually, intralymphatically,[56] orally, or nasally. This article discusses only subcutaneous immunotherapy (SCIT) and sublingual immunotherapy (SLIT). The mechanism of immunotherapy is not known precisely, but likely depends on changes in T-helper lymphocytes down-regulating inflammation and shifting the inflammatory mediator profile toward nonallergic.

#### SCIT

Subcutaneous immunotherapy, or allergy desensitization shots, involves injecting the allergens to which the patient is sensitized (allergic) into the subcutaneous tissue (usually of the arm). There are 2 phases of SCIT: escalation and maintenance. During escalation, the patient is started at a sufficiently dilute dose to be safe and each subsequent shot contains a higher amount of allergen. Through serial shots provided once or twice a week, the amount of allergen is increased several thousand fold. Once a tolerated dose in the effective range is established, maintenance therapy involves giving the same dose at regular intervals. Gradually the time between shots is increased to monthly. The duration of maintenance therapy is generally 3 to 5 years and most patients can discontinue and retain the clinical benefit, although there is significant individual variation.[55]

Randomized controlled trials and meta-analyses have supported efficacy for SCIT in single-antigen studies[57]; however, most patients with allergic rhinitis have multiple sensitivities and are desensitized using combined allergens. SCIT exposes allergic patients to higher than natural exposures of allergen and each shot poses the risk of triggering anaphylaxis. Time, expense, and anaphylactic risk of immunotherapy need to be considered in selecting and counseling patients. Immunotherapy is reserved for moderate and severe allergic rhinitis not controlled easily with other measures.

### SLIT

Sublingual immunotherapy is performed by placing drops of allergen extract under the tongue. Holding the extract under the tongue seems to allow the allergens to be taken up into the regional lymphatics. Multiple studies using different allergens, techniques (spit or swallow), frequencies, durations, and doses have been published, and meta-analyses have suggested effectiveness, although none of the variables is agreed on.[58] Initial industry-sponsored studies looking at sublingual therapy for grass allergy have also shown efficacy and safety,[59,60] although SLIT is not approved by the Food and Drug Administration. While initial studies showed excellent safety, some reports of systemic reactions have been presented, especially after the first dose.[61] Many sublingual protocols recommend daily drops given at home, and controversy exists as to level of safety expected for home therapy treating a nonlethal disease. Interestingly, systemic allergic reactions treated with epinephrine also appear in the placebo arms of some studies. The combination of safety, efficacy, and convenience make SLIT a compelling option. In the author's opinion, some of the controversy over SLIT may be biased by its potential socioeconomic impact.

### SUMMARY

Facial plastic surgeons should develop expertise in nasal anatomy and pathophysiology to address functional and aesthetic consequences of nasal surgery. One area where allergic rhinitis may impact plastic surgery outcomes is aesthetic rhinoplasty. Aesthetic rhinoplasty can alter nasal function by narrowing the nasal valve. Nasal obstruction is more likely in patients with allergic rhinitis, as they have intermittent or persistent turbinate swelling. Identifying and managing allergic rhinitis in patients considering cosmetic nasal surgery should lead to better surgical outcomes and may inform decisions on the functional consequences of nasal surgery. Allergic rhinitis is primarily a clinical diagnosis and allergy testing is complementary. Allergy testing alone should not be relied on for screening, as the false positive rate is likely unacceptable. Allergic rhinitis

is manageable in most individuals through choices of pharmacotherapy, environmental control, and allergen immunotherapy. There may be a role for turbinate reduction, nasal valve surgery, and septoplasty in selected patients with allergic rhinitis refractory to nonsurgical management. The diagnosis and management of allergic rhinitis should assist in better selection, counseling, and outcomes for patients considering aesthetic nasal surgery.

## REFERENCES

1. Marple BF, Fornadley JA, Patel AA, et al. Keys to successful management of patients with allergic rhinitis: focus on patient confidence, compliance, and satisfaction. Otolaryngol Head Neck Surg 2007;136(Suppl 6):S107–24.
2. Krouse JH, Brown RW, Fineman SM, et al. Asthma and the unified airway. Otolaryngol Head Neck Surg 2007;136(Suppl 5):S75–106.
3. Bousquet J, Khaltaev N, Cruz AA, et al. Allergic Rhinitis and its Impact on Asthma (ARIA) 2008 update (in collaboration with the World Health Organization, GA(2)LEN and AllerGen). Allergy 2008; 63(Suppl 86):8–160.
4. Ober C, Hoffjan S. Asthma genetics 2006: the long and winding road to gene discovery. Genes Immun 2006;7(2):95–100.
5. Holloway JW, Yang IA, Holgate ST. Genetics of allergic disease. J Allergy Clin Immunol 2010; 125(2 Suppl 2):S81–94.
6. Smith FJ, Irvine AD, Terron-Kwiatkowski A, et al. Loss-of-function mutations in the gene encoding filaggrin cause ichthyosis vulgaris. Nat Genet 2006; 38(3):337–42.
7. Kay AB. Allergy and allergic diseases. Second of two parts. N Engl J Med 2001;344(2):109–13.
8. Lieberman P. The basics of histamine biology. Ann Allergy Asthma Immunol 2011;106(Suppl 2):S2–5.
9. Han D, Wang C, Lou W, et al. Allergen-specific IL-10-secreting type I T regulatory cells, but not CD4(+)CD25(+)Foxp3(+) T cells, are decreased in peripheral blood of patients with persistent allergic rhinitis. Clin Immunol 2010;136(2):292–301.
10. Ronmark E, Bjerg A, Perzanowski M, et al. Major increase in allergic sensitization in schoolchildren from 1996 to 2006 in northern Sweden. J Allergy Clin Immunol 2009;124(2):357–63, e351–5.
11. Pleis JR, Ward BW, Lucas JW. Summary health statistics for U.S. adults: National Health Interview Survey, 2009. National Center for Health Statistics. Vital Health Stat 2010;10(249). Available at: http://www.cdc.gov/nchs/data/series/sr_10/sr10_249.pdf. Accessed April 24, 2011.
12. Bloom B, Cohen RA, Freeman G. Summary health statistics for U.S. children: National Health Interview

Survey, 2009. National Center for Health Statistics. Vital Health Stat 2010;10(247). Available at: http://www.cdc.gov/nchs/data/series/sr_10/sr10_247.pdf. Accessed April 24, 2011.

13. Meltzer EO, Bukstein DA. The economic impact of allergic rhinitis and current guidelines for treatment. Ann Allergy Asthma Immunol 2011;106(Suppl 2): S12–6.

14. Ker J, Hartert TV. The atopic march: what's the evidence? Ann Allergy Asthma Immunol 2009; 103(4):282–9.

15. Bach JF. The effect of infections on susceptibility to autoimmune and allergic diseases. N Engl J Med 2002;347(12):911–20.

16. Okada H, Kuhn C, Feillet H, et al. The 'hygiene hypothesis' for autoimmune and allergic diseases: an update. Clin Exp Immunol 2010;160(1):1–9.

17. Doyle WJ, Skoner DP, Seroky JT, et al. Reproducibility of the effects of intranasal ragweed challenges in allergic subjects. Ann Allergy Asthma Immunol 1995;74(2):171–6.

18. Abraham CM, Ownby DR, Peterson EL, et al. The relationship between seroatopy and symptoms of either allergic rhinitis or asthma. J Allergy Clin Immunol 2007;119(5):1099–104.

19. Bousquet J, Neukirch F, Bousquet PJ, et al. Severity and impairment of allergic rhinitis in patients consulting in primary care. J Allergy Clin Immunol 2006; 117(1):158–62.

20. Skadhauge LR, Christensen K, Kyvik KO, et al. Genetic and environmental influence on asthma: a population-based study of 11,688 Danish twin pairs. Eur Respir J 1999;13(1):8–14.

21. Wallace DV, Dykewicz MS, Bernstein DI, et al. The diagnosis and management of rhinitis: an updated practice parameter. J Allergy Clin Immunol 2008; 122(Suppl 2):S1–84.

22. Slavin RG. Allergy is not a significant cause of nasal polyps. Arch Otolaryngol Head Neck Surg 1992; 118(3):343.

23. Franzooo CB, Burkhalter NW. The patient with allergies. Med Clin North Am 2010;94(5):891–902.

24. Krouse JH, Dworkin JP, Carron MA, et al. Baseline laryngeal effects among individuals with dust mite allergy. Otolaryngol Head Neck Surg 2008;139(1): 149–51.

25. Arbes SJ Jr, Gergen PJ, Elliott L, et al. Prevalences of positive skin test responses to 10 common allergens in the US population: results from the third National Health and Nutrition Examination Survey. J Allergy Clin Immunol 2005;116(2): 377–83.

26. Tschopp JM, Sistek D, Schindler C, et al. Current allergic asthma and rhinitis: diagnostic efficiency of three commonly used atopic markers (IgE, skin prick tests, and Phadiatop). Results from 8329 randomized adults from the SAPALDIA Study. Swiss Study on Air Pollution and Lung Diseases in Adults. Allergy 1998;53(6):608–13.

27. Noon L. Prophylactic inoculation against hayfever. Lancet 1911;1:1572–3.

28. Guidelines for the Diagnosis and Management of Food Allergy. 2010. Available at: http://www.niaid.nih.gov/topics/foodallergy/clinical/Pages/default.aspx. Accessed November 14, 2010.

29. Malm L, Gerth van Wijk R, Bachert C. Guidelines for nasal provocations with aspects on nasal patency, airflow, and airflow resistance. International Committee on Objective Assessment of the Nasal Airways, International Rhinologic Society. Rhinology 2000;38(1):1–6.

30. Krouse JH, Mabry RL. Skin testing for inhalant allergy 2003: current strategies. Otolaryngol Head Neck Surg 2003;129(Suppl 4):S33–49.

31. Nelson HS, Oppenheimer J, Buchmeier A, et al. An assessment of the role of intradermal skin testing in the diagnosis of clinically relevant allergy to timothy grass. J Allergy Clin Immunol 1996;97(6): 1193–201.

32. Hamilton RG. Clinical laboratory assessment of immediate-type hypersensitivity. J Allergy Clin Immunol 2010;125(2 Suppl 2):S284–96.

33. Sampson HA. Food allergy—accurately identifying clinical reactivity. Allergy 2005;60(Suppl 79):19–24.

34. Graif Y, Goldberg A, Tamir R, et al. Skin test results and self-reported symptom severity in allergic rhinitis: the role of psychological factors. Clin Exp Allergy 2006;36(12):1532–7.

35. Barboo RA, Halonen M, Lebowitz M, et al. Distribution of IgE in a community population sample: correlations with age, sex, and allergen skin test reactivity. J Allergy Clin Immunol 1981;68(2):106–11.

36. Day JH, Briscoe M, Rafeiro E, et al. Comparative onset of action and symptom relief with cetirizine, loratadine, or placebo in an environmental exposure unit in subjects with seasonal allergic rhinitis: confirmation of a test system. Ann Allergy Asthma Immunol 2001;87(6):474–81.

37. Howarth PH, Stern MA, Roi L, et al. Double-blind, placebo-controlled study comparing the efficacy and safety of fexofenadine hydrochloride (120 and 180 mg once daily) and cetirizine in seasonal allergic rhinitis. J Allergy Clin Immunol 1999; 104(5):927–33.

38. Stubner P, Zieglmayer R, Horak F. A direct comparison of the efficacy of antihistamines in SAR and PAR: randomised, placebo-controlled studies with levocetirizine and loratadine using an environmental exposure unit—the Vienna Challenge Chamber (VCC). Curr Med Res Opin 2004;20(6): 891–902.

39. Ratner PH, Hampel F, Van Bavel J, et al. Combination therapy with azelastine hydrochloride nasal spray and fluticasone propionate nasal spray in the

treatment of patients with seasonal allergic rhinitis. Ann Allergy Asthma Immunol 2008;100(1):74–81.

40. Pullerits T, Praks L, Ristioja V, et al. Comparison of a nasal glucocorticoid, antileukotriene, and a combination of antileukotriene and antihistamine in the treatment of seasonal allergic rhinitis. J Allergy Clin Immunol 2002;109(6):949–55.

41. Grootendorst DC, Dahlen SE, Van Den Bos JW, et al. Benefits of high altitude allergen avoidance in atopic adolescents with moderate to severe asthma, over and above treatment with high dose inhaled steroids. Clin Exp Allergy 2001;31(3):400–8.

42. Frederick JM, Warner JO, Jessop WJ, et al. Effect of a bed covering system in children with asthma and house dust mite hypersensitivity. Eur Respir J 1997;10(2):361–6.

43. Tovey ER, Marks GB, Matthews M, et al. Changes in mite allergen Der p I in house dust following spraying with a tannic acid/acaricide solution. Clin Exp Allergy 1992;22(1):67–74.

44. Chang JH, Becker A, Ferguson A, et al. Effect of application of benzyl benzoate on house dust mite allergen levels. Ann Allergy Asthma Immunol 1996; 77(3):187–90.

45. Munir AK, Einarsson R, Dreborg SK. Vacuum cleaning decreases the levels of mite allergens in house dust. Pediatr Allergy Immunol 1993;4(3):136–43.

46. Green R, Simpson A, Custovic A, et al. The effect of air filtration on airborne dog allergen. Allergy 1999; 54(5):484–8.

47. Choi SY, Lee IY, Sohn JH, et al. Optimal conditions for the removal of house dust mite, dog dander, and pollen allergens using mechanical laundry. Ann Allergy Asthma Immunol 2008; 100(6):583–8.

48. de Blay F, Chapman MD, Platts-Mills TA. Airborne cat allergen (Fel d I). Environmental control with the cat in situ. Am Rev Respir Dis 1991;143(6): 1334–9.

49. Nageotte C, Park M, Havstad S, et al. Duration of airborne Fel d 1 reduction after cat washing. J Allergy Clin Immunol 2006;118(2):521–2.

50. Terreehorst I, Hak E, Oosting AJ, et al. Evaluation of impermeable covers for bedding in patients with allergic rhinitis. N Engl J Med 2003;349(3):237–46.

51. Sheikh A, Hurwitz B, Nurmatov U, et al. House dust mite avoidance measures for perennial allergic rhinitis. Cochrane Database Syst Rev 2010;7: CD001563.

52. Gunhan K, Unlu H, Yuceturk AV, et al. Intranasal steroids or radiofrequency turbinoplasty in persistent allergic rhinitis: effects on quality of life and objective parameters. Eur Arch Otorhinolaryngol 2011;268(6):845–50.

53. Mori S, Fujieda S, Yamada T, et al. Long-term effect of submucous turbinectomy in patients with perennial allergic rhinitis. Laryngoscope 2002;112(5):865–9.

54. Lin HC, Lin PW, Su CY, et al. Radiofrequency for the treatment of allergic rhinitis refractory to medical therapy. Laryngoscope 2003;113(4):673–8.

55. Osguthorpe JD. Immunotherapy. Curr Opin Otolaryngol Head Neck Surg 2010;18(3):206–12.

56. Martinez-Gomez JM, Johansen P, Erdmann I, et al. Intralymphatic injections as a new administration route for allergen-specific immunotherapy. Int Arch Allergy Immunol 2009;150(1):59–65.

57. Calderon MA, Alves B, Jacobson M, et al. Allergen injection immunotherapy for seasonal allergic rhinitis. Cochrane Database Syst Rev 2007;1:CD001936.

58. Leatherman BD, Owen S, Parker M, et al. Sublingual immunotherapy: past, present, paradigm for the future? A review of the literature. Otolaryngol Head Neck Surg 2007;136(Suppl 3):S1–20.

59. Halken S, Agertoft L, Seidenberg J, et al. Five-grass pollen 300IR SLIT tablets: efficacy and safety in children and adolescents. Pediatr Allergy Immunol 2010;21(6):970–6.

60. Wahn U, Tabar A, Kuna P, et al. Efficacy and safety of 5-grass-pollen sublingual immunotherapy tablets in pediatric allergic rhinoconjunctivitis. J Allergy Clin Immunol 2009;123(1):160–6, e163.

61. de Groot H, Bijl A. Anaphylactic reaction after the first dose of sublingual immunotherapy with grass pollen tablet. Allergy 2009;64(6):963–4.

# Nonallergic Rhinitis

Stephanie A. Joe, MD

## KEYWORDS

- Nonallergic rhinitis • Vasomotor rhinitis • Chronic rhinitis
- Irritant rhinitis • Idiopathic rhinitis

---

### Key Points

- A patient with rhinitis symptoms should be fully evaluated from a rhinologic standpoint before nasal surgery is undertaken.
- If diagnosed with rhinitis, the patient should be aware that his or her complaints may not be improved with surgery alone; maintenance medical therapy may be required postoperatively.
- Although a common reason for nonallergic rhinitis (NAR), vasomotor rhinitis is a diagnosis of exclusion.
- Systemic diseases and local factors can contribute to NAR and should be recognized by the facial plastic surgeon caring for her or his patients.
- Patient education and awareness of symptom triggers are key factors in the management of NAR.
- Although there are few medications specifically for NAR, it can usually be reasonably managed with a combination of medical therapy and avoidance measures.
- Allergic rhinitis (AR) and NAR may coexist in the same patient. The facial plastic surgeon should be ready to address these entities.

---

An estimated 17 to 19 million Americans are affected by NAR.[1,2] Women seem to be more affected by rhinitis, with 70% of women aged 50 to 64 experiencing some form of rhinitis during a 1-year period.[3,4] Chronic rhinitis symptoms often interfere with school and/or work performance, and a lack of productivity is worsened by the need for frequent doctor visits. In a recent survey of rhinitis patients, 25% noted restricting their choice of occupation or residence to reduce their symptoms.[5] In addition, medications—although usually helpful—may elicit undesirable side effects such as drowsiness, epistaxis, palpitations, and nasal dryness, which compound the overall impact of NAR.[6]

NAR and AR have similar presentations, manifestations, treatments, and impacts on school and work performance. Thus, statistics for AR can be used to infer the economic impact of NAR.

In many instances, AR and NAR are often indistinguishable and co-exist.[1,2] Twenty to 40 million Americans are affected by AR, and the direct costs for doctor visits and medication expenses are at least $1.9 billion annually. The cost of lost productivity approaches $3.8 billion annually.[7]

Of the patients who present to the otolaryngologist's office, 50% are diagnosed with a form of NAR, and the rest are diagnosed with AR.[1,8] In a survey of 975 patients visiting allergists' offices for chronic rhinitis, the National Classification Task Force found that 43% were diagnosed with pure AR, 23% with NAR, and 34% with mixed AR and NAR. Thus, 57% of chronic rhinitis patients have some component of NAR.[9]

Despite the health care burden of NAR, defining it is difficult. Symptom presentation is nonspecific, and patients may present in a variety of ways. Historically, vasomotor rhinitis was the term used

Financial disclosure: The author is a consultant for Gyrus ENT, an Olympus company.
Department of Otolaryngology–Head and Neck Surgery (MC 648), University of Illinois at Chicago, 1855 West Taylor Street, Room 2.42, Chicago, IL 60612, USA
E-mail address: sjoe@uic.edu

facialplastic.theclinics.com

to describe chronic, NAR; however, motor nerve or vascular dysfunction has not been well-described.[8,10] Other terms used include perennial rhinitis, idiopathic rhinitis, perennial NAR, and nonallergic, noninfectious perennial rhinitis.[2,8,11,12] Nonallergic rhinitis is the term used in this article to describe the various forms of the symptom complex of nasal congestion, obstruction, intermittent rhinorrhea as well as occasional itching and sneezing unrelated to an identifable allergen sensitivity by skin or serum testing.

In many cases of NAR, treatment is often indiscriminate, with varied responses seen among patients. The results are often unsatisfactory and frustrating for both the physician and the patient. Because there have been no unifying criteria for this broad class of problems, further investigation and work-up are generally abandoned by many clinicians, especially since there are no clear diagnostic tests. This article will review a uniform way to describe nonallergic rhinitis in its various forms. The insights into it pathophysiology is briefly reviewed. A classification scheme for the different forms is provided. This is followed by descriptions of the diagnosis, evaluation and management of NAR.

## INSIGHTS INTO THE PATHOPHYSIOLOGY OF NAR

Attempting to understand the pathophysiology of NAR requires an appreciation of nasal function. The upper and lower respiratory tracts are lined with pseudostratified ciliated columnar epithelium, which contains goblet cells, ciliated cells, and basal cells. This lining serves in the important regulatory functions for the nose, including the filtration and humdification of inspired air, temperature regulation, olfaction, and preparation of the inspired air for the lower airways.

The mucosa produces mucus secretions that provide lubrication. Additionally, these secretions contain lysozyme, glycoproteins, lactoferrin, and secretory immunoglobulin A, providing protection for the airway. The cilia propel the mucous blanket and their trapped contents toward the natural sinus ostia and toward the nasopharynx.[13]

The mucosa has a rich vascular supply with abundant venous sinusoids. The nasal cycle is comprised of a normal physiologic phenomenon during which time the nasal mucosa will alternately engorge and decongest. This is regulated by the autonomic nervous system, which controls the vasculature as well as glandular secretions.[8,13]

Sensation primarily originates from the trigeminal nerve. Afferent ethmoidal nerves provide sensory innervation to the epithelium, vessels, and glands. Unspecified afferent sensory nerves called C-fibers react to pain and changes in temperature and osmolarity; they are the most relevant type of sensory fibers in NAR. These sensory fibers are stimulated by inflammatory mediators such as histamine and bradykinin and are involved in centrally mediated reflexes. Once stimulated, C-fibers depolarize, leading to increased vascular permeability and submucosal gland release. There is also acute stimulation of nasal mucosal endothelial cells and epithelial cells, with the resultant sensation of itching and/or burning, and the production of mucoid rhinorrhea.[8]

The sympathetic portion of the autonomic nervous system comprises 50% of the efferent nasal reflex arc, which causes vasoconstriction of the nasal vasculature. The parasympathetic nerves form the other half of the efferent nasal reflex arc, with relaxation of the blood vessels and stimulation of the serous glands of the nasal mucosa. Notably, unilateral stimulation of the efferent reflex arc leads to a bilateral response.[8,10,13]

In essence, a derangement of any component of the nasal mucosa may lead to the symptoms of NAR. The nonspecific and variable symptoms of NAR are confounding; this compounds the difficult task of identifying the exact pathophysiologic source. Various possible etiologies for NAR have been investigated:

1. Inflammation
2. Hyperreactivity of the parasympathetic limb of the autonomic nervous system and/or hyporeactivity of the sympathetic arm
3. Glandular hyper-reactivity
4. Hypersensitivity of the sensory input via by C-fibers.

Recent research on patients with NAR has begun to evaluate the role of mucosal immunoglobulin E (IgE) and inflammatory cell production.[14] A subgroup of patients with NAR has been found to demonstrate an increased local prodcution of IgE upon nasal provocation testing.[15] A separate study indicates that a subgroup of NAR patients, who by definition are not systemtically atopic, may display a local allergic disease pathway.[16] This group could possibly be those classically described as possessing NAR with eosinophilia syndrome, or NARES.

In the case of potential autonomic problems, hyper-responsiveness of the afferent sensory limb leads to an exaggerated efferent response with resultant oversecretion of mucus and increased nasal congestion due to capillary plasma exudation. The same symptoms are seen with normal afferent input and a hyper-reactive efferent arc. Less commonly, an intrinsic epithelial problem or a problem with central nervous system regulation can be the source of disordered responsiveness. Unfortunately, given the complex interaction of sinonasal mucosal regulation, it has been difficult to develop an accurate study model.[10,17]

The inhalation of irritants is linked to the stimulation of the C-fibers, afferent sensory nerves in nasal mucosa, which innervate the epithelium, vessels, and glands. This results in the activation of the parasympathetic nerves and subsequent sneezing, rhinorrhea, and congestion. This reaction may be induced by histamine and possibly lead to an immunomodulatory response and local cellular events.[18] Glandular hypersecretion can also occur independent of sensory nerve stimulation, as has been shown in methacholine challenge tests.[12,19] Such findings indicate increased mucosal sensitivity and reactivity in patients with NAR.

Nasal provocation testing using various stimulants has been performed in attempts to characterize NAR. In addition to methacholine, histamine, cold dry air, and capsaicin have all been studied. However, no one study model has provided definitive information regarding the physiologic mechanisms involved in NAR. In many of the studies, the stimulant evaluated induced nasal symptoms greater than seen in controls, but symptom response often overlapped with those patients diagnosed AR. Unfortunately, studies exist with contrary results. Additionally, comparison between studies is difficult, as study methods have not been uniform. Furthermore, provocation studies have shown that upon stimulation, multiple reactions may occur simultaneously (eg, release of inflammatory mediators as well as an exagerrated autonomic response). As a result, there are many examples of how to study the many facets of the pathophysiology of NAR, but there is currently no specific model.[9,12,19,26]

## TYPES OF NAR
### NARES

NARES was first described in 1981.[27] Patients were described as having perennial nasal complaints, rhinorrhea, epiphora, sneezing, and pruritis typical for AR. Cytologic examination of nasal secretions showed marked eosinophilia. However, the patients lacked immunologic reaction to common inhalant allergens. Most of the patients denied a specific trigger, although some reported reactions to weather changes, odors, or chemical irritants. Other studies demonstrated that mast cells, IgE-positive cells, and eosinophils are increased in the nasal mucosa of both AR

and NAR patients, possiby as a consequence of localized IgE-mediated reactions. In these patients, epithelial damage was seen in the presence of high local eosinophil counts. Nasal neural dysfunction has also been described to contribute to the symptomatology in NARES-type patients.[14,28]

### Hormone-Related Rhinitis

Rhinitis during pregnancy is a probably one of the best known forms of NAR. Rhinorrhea and congestion are prominent, and a review of the patient's history frequently elicits a prior history of chronic rhinitis, either allergic or nonallergic.[29] The etiology of this condition is considered to be due in part to direct effects on the nasal mucosa from changes in estrogen, progesterone, prolactin, and placental growth hormone levels.[30,31] Vascular changes and physiologic expansion of circulating blood volume may also contribute to increased nasal vascular pooling and progesterone-induced vascular smooth muscle relaxation.[1,30]

Hormones may act directly on the nasal mucosa, causing mucus gland hyper-reactivity and increased rhinorrhea.[1] As such, nasal symptoms may be associated with systemic conditions that result from hormone imbalance such as hypothyroidism and acromegaly.[8] Rhinitis may arise as a result of changing blood hormone concentrations during puberty. Fluctuating serum hormone levels during menstruation and perimenopause are also associated with nasal symptoms.[32]

### Medication-Associated Rhinitis

Rhinitis is a common adverse effect of the chronic use decongestant medications. Obtaining a patient history about medication overuse of topical nasal decongestants and cocaine abuse is critical. Frequent or prolonged use can result in rebound congestion that induces dependency on medication use for relief of nasal airway mucosal obstruction.

Rhinitis is an adverse effect of a myriad of other medications. Medications that affect the vasculature for the treatment of hypertension and cardiac conditions can also affect the nasal mucosa. The suspected patient should be queried about the use of beta-blockers, angiotensin-converting enzyme inhibitors, alpha-blockers, and vasodilators. As mentioned earlier, hormones are associated with nasal symptoms, so a history of the use of hormone replacement and oral contraceptives should also be sought. Psychotropic agents are also associated with congestion (eg, thioridazine, amitriptyline, perphenazine). The use of selective seritonin reuptake inhibitors may be associated with rhinitis-type adverse effects as well. Nonsteroidal anti-inflammatory medications are well known for their potential association with rhinosinusitis, sinonasal polyps, and asthma.[8,10]

### Irritant Rhinitis

The production of profuse, mucoid rhinorrhea is known to be stimulated by cold, dry air.[22,33] Facial pressure and headaches as well as nasal symptoms can be brought on by altitude shifts in some patients such as pilots and flight attendants. Alterations in barometric pressure and temperature can be other inciting causes of this form of NAR.

Gustatory rhinitis occurs when the ingestion of foods leads to mucoid or watery rhinorrhea that lasts for as long as the food is ingested.[1,34] Hot, spicy foods are a common culprit, but sometimes just the act of eating can lead to runny nose. Other nasal symptoms are often absent; however, sweating and epiphora may accompany the reaction. The likely pathophysiologic mechanism is the stimulation of afferent sensory nerves with resultant activation of the parasympathetic nerves supplying the nasal mucosal and sweat glands.[34]

Tobacco smoke, perfumes, floral fragrances, and cleaning chemicals produce annoyance reactions and are known triggers in patients with a heightened sense of olfaction. Also, some foods and alcohol are triggers for many patients. Patients are often sensitive to multiple irritants that are part of their environment. Air pollution and ozone levels are discussed daily in susceptible areas and times of the year.[1]

### Occupational Forms of Rhinitis

The occupational form of rhinitis is a special form of irritant rhinitis that represents a complex form of inhalant-induced rhinitis. Various types of chemical exposure have been classifeid by Baraniuk and Kaliner and consist of immunologic, annoyance, irritational, and corrosive forms.[35] Airway reactions can occur with suprathreshold exposure to chemicals and fumes in the workplace. Oftentimes, reactions are a result of exposure to respiratory inhalant irritants beyond threshold levels. Paint fumes, formaldehyde, oxides of nitrogen, and toluene are also examples of this problem.

Although the pathophysiology is not well understood, there is support that many forms of irritant rhinitis are mediated by neurogenic mechanisms, particularly those that are related to chemical exposures. Neurogenic inflammation is considered a pathway model in chemical sensitivity syndromes, including some forms of chronic rhinitis and asthma. As discussed earlier, the proposed mechanism is the stimulation of irritant receptors on sensory nerves (ie, C-fibers), which induces neuropeptide mediator release. The mediator release then produces vasodilation and edema associated with inflammation independent of immune-mediated inflammation.[36,37]

Unfortunately, along with typical NAR symptoms, victims of occupational rhinitis may also develop nasal mucosal hyper-reactivity, and problems with an impaired sense of smell, nosebleeds, nasal crusting, and reduced mucociliary function.[38] Nasal and oral mucosal contact with high concentrations of soluble chemical gases can cause inflammation, burns and ulcerations, as well as skin and eye reactions. Examples of such corrosive reactions include those associated with exposures to ammonium, chloride, hydrochloric acid, vinyl chloride, organophosphates, and acrylamide.[1]

The prevalence of occupational rhinitis is estimated to be 5% to 15%. Nonallergic forms should be differentiated from occupationally induced allergic or immunologic rhinitis.[39] Immunologic aeroallergens associated with rhinitis in the workplace include animal proteins, wheat, latex, pyrethrum in the insecticide and garden industries, acid anhydrides in the adhesive industry, and toluene in auto body spray paints. As such, a detailed workplace history is essential.

### Idiopathic

A diagnosis of idiopathic or vasomotor rhinitis is given when other identifiable causes of NAR have been excluded. Unfortunately, it is the most common form of NAR. Speculated as an entity more than 50 years ago, vasomotor rhinitis was historically considered to be due to an imbalance of the autonomic nerve supply to the nasal mucosa.[2,4,11] Studies since then have demonstrated a possible relationship between vasomotor rhinitis and autonomic nervous system dysfunction. Hypoactivity of the sympathetic nervous system relative to the parasympathetic nervous system results in the diversity of local and systemic symptoms that may be seen in vasomotor rhinitis and autonomic dysfunction.[40,41]

### Associated Local and Systemic Problems

Local factors affecting the nose can result in nasal symptoms. Anatomic findings such as the presence of a septal deviation or nasal valve collapse affect nasal airflow and may give a sense of congestion. Hypertrophic turbinates may be a result of chronic rhinitis but also cause physical alterations in the nasal airway. The presence of a septal perforation alters the natural lamellar airflow of the nasal cavities and may be perceived as congestion or obstruction by the patient.

The nasal symptoms that result from obstruction from inflammatory disease such as polyps or neoplasms are sometimes diagnosed as rhinitis or sinus problems before the correct diagnosis is made. Rhinitis may be the first sign of inflammatory sinonasal disease or infection. Systemic problems such as autoimmune disorders or vasculitides such as Sjogren syndrome, lupus, sacoidosis, Wegener syndrome, and Churg-straus syndrome are associated with chronic rhinitis. Congenital problems associated with ciliary dysmotility must also be kept in mind. Cystic fibrosis is also part of the differential diagnosis in chronic rhinitis.[10]

## HISTORY AND DIAGNOSIS OF NAR

A thorough history of sinonasal complaints often provides the practitioner with the suspicions for the diagnosis of NAR. In addition to acquiring a complete patient history, the practitioner should include extensive questioning with regard to the pattern and timing of symptoms, exacerbating and relieving factors, and environmental triggers. A history indicative of NAR in a healthy patient includes age of onset in mid-30s, a lack of seasonal symptom exacerbation, and negative family history for allergies. A history of symptom exacerbation around perfumes or strong odors lends further support.

However, the practitioner should be aware that many patients may suffer with both AR and NAR. The presence of one form of rhinitis may compound the coexistent condition, resulting in severe and often persistent symptoms. Also, multiple systemic conditions may contribute or result in NAR as mentioned previously. With these possibilities in mind, the practitioner obtaining the history must also pay attention to the patient's past medical history and medication history.

A comprehensive head and neck examination includes the findings as seen on nasal endoscopy. The mucosa is usually boggy and edematous with clear mucoid secretions. Mucosal injection and lymphoid hyperplasia involving the tonsils, adenoids, and base of the tongue may be seen to varying degrees. Areas of blanched mucosa surrounding prominent vessels have been reported in chemical exposures.[42] The presence of inflammation and purulent discharge from the middle meatus and sphenoethmoid recess indicate active infection. Polyps are an indication of chronic inflammation and obstruction. Atrophy

of the mucosa is seen in cases of aging, prior surgery, and drug abuse. Anatomic obstruction can be diagnosed with the presences of septal deviation, hypertrophic turbinates, and choanal stenosis or atresia. Nasal valve collapse is often overlooked when patients complain of nasal obstruction. The presence of a septal perforation with crusting and epistaxis can be associated with similar symptoms. Examination of the nasal cavity and nasopharynx also helps identify adenoid hypertrophy or unusual mucosal lesions suggestive of sarcoidosis or Wegener syndrome.

Testing for inhalant allergies should be part of the diagnostic work-up in NAR. This can be accomplished via skin or serum testing for specific IgE antibodies to local allergens. Information on cell types and the presence of inflammation is obtained by performing cytologic examination of nasal secretions. Microscopic examination revealing a high power field of 5 to 25 eosinophils in the absence of atopy is compatible with a diagnosis of NARES.[27]

As mentioned earlier, some forms of chronic rhinitis have also been associated with smell impairment.[43] As such, validated smell testing can be a useful addition in the diagnostic work-up and management of patients with NAR. When available, measurements with acoustic rhinometry or rhinomanometry can provide information regarding nasal patency and responses to provocation testing.[44,45]

Imaging with plain radiographs or computed tomography (CT) scanning is not particularly useful in uncomplicated rhinitis, especially after initial nasal endoscopy is performed. However, CT scans may be useful for evaluating sinonasal inflammatory disease, anatomic obstruction such as the presence of a concha bullosa or polups, skull base defects, and cerebrospinal fluid rhinorrhea. Magnetic resonance imaging would be useful when a neoplasm is suspected.

## TREATMENT OF NAR
### Avoidance

Patient education is the most important factor in the treatment of NAR. Frequently, patients cannot immediately recall the specific trigger that incites their symptoms, but a thorough and accurate history can often elucidate the cause of an individual's problem and provides information for the patient. With this knowledge, the patient can take an active role in his or her health care and control his or her environment. Avoidance of inciting factors such as perfumes, tobacco smoke, cleaning supplies, and certain foods or wines can usually be accomplished without great difficulty.

If a change in environment is not feasible, occupational exposures can be eliminated by donning masks and protective coverings. The associated medications can be discontinued or changed. Unfortunately, in many circumstances, exposure to inciting triggers cannot be avoided; no substitute exists for an essential medication, or avoidance measures are not enough to control symptoms. In these cases, medical therapy can be used to supplement the control the symptoms of NAR. The clinician must remember that coexistent AR may complicate the diagnosis and treatment of NAR.

## MEDICAL THERAPY FOR NAR
### Topical Nasal Steroids

Topical nasal steroids decrease neutrophil and eosinophil chemotaxis, reduce mast cell and basophil mediator release, and result in decreased mucosal edema and local inflammation.[46] Although the pathophysiology of NAR is incompletely understood, topical nasal steroids are widely used for the treatment of NAR and are noted to be effective.

Optimal medication administration requires propelling the medications into the nasal cavity. Approximately 20% of intranasal steroid preparations are absorbed into the nasal mucosa; the most of the remaining 80% are swallowed and undergo first-pass hepatic metabolism in the portal circulation. Pointing the spray nozzle upward and away from the nasal septum is recommended. Topical steroids are generally tolerated quite well, and adverse effects are infrequently encountered. The most commonly reported adverse effects include anterior septal irritation, nasal dryness and crusts, epistaxis, throat irritation, and headaches. Systemic adverse effects are quite rare. Since the effectiveness of nasal steroids requires contact with the nasal mucosa, anatomic obstruction as well as obstruction from polyps and turbinate hypertrophy may prevent topical steroids from reaching their destination.

Given the findings of eosinophils and inflammation on nasal cytology, NARES is likely to respond well to topical nasal steroids.[1] Fluticasone propionate, beclomethasone, and budesonide are currently the only topical steroids preparations with a US Food and Drug Administration (FDA) indication for treating NAR.[47] Also, budesonide is currently the only topical nasal steroid that has a pregnancy category of B, whereas all others are category C.[48] It is recommended that these medications are used on a daily basis for maximum benefit, and a trial should be given for a minimum 6 weeks.

### Antihistamines

Azelastine is a topical nasal antihistamine that is approved for use in both AR and NAR. Just like oral antihistamines, azelastine is an H1-receptor antagonist. In addition, studies show that it inhibits the synthesis of leukotrienes, kinins, and cytokines. It also inhibits the expression of intercellular adhesion molecules and the generation of superoxide free radicals. These anti-inflammatory effects, which are unrelated to H1-receptor antagonism, allow azelastine to provide relief in NARES and vasomotor rhinitis. This is felt by the patient as the relief of obstruction and decreased nasal symptoms, mucosal edema, and decreased amounts of rhinorrhea.[49,50] This medication is generally well tolerated with a low discontinuation rate of 2.3%.[51] Azelastine is a reasonable consideration in those patients with mixed AR and NAR.

Oral antihistamines tend to have a limited role in treating NAR; however, they may be beneficial for patients with NAR who also have sneezing as a component of their symptom complex.[52] Adverse effects for both oral and nasal antihistamines are related to their anticholinergic properties.[53]

### Anticholinergic Nasal Spray

This class of medications is useful in the management of bothersome rhinorrhea as can be seen in NAR. The nasal preparation, ipratropium bromide, acts locally to block parasympathetic input to the nasal mucosal glands. The 0.03% strength is approved by the FDA for treating AR and NAR. Initially, 2 sprays are given 3 times a day. Symptom control should become apparent within 1 week. When symptoms abate, the dosing can be lowered by 1 spray at a time. One spray 2 times daily is the lowest recommended maintenance dose. It can be used in children as young as 6 years of age. For pregnant women, it carries a class B label. The use of intranasal ipratropium may be associated with local side effects such as nasal dryness and epistaxis. These problems are usually tolerable and their incidence decreased with continued use of the medication or dosage adjustment.[54,55]

### Nasal Saline

Frequent use of nasal saline spray mists throughout the day and the daily use of nasal saline irrigations are useful in managing the symptoms of NAR. This therapy serves to cleanse the nose of irritants, improve mucociliary clearance, and aid in the management of mucoid secretions.

## THE ROLE OF SURGERY IN NAR

As mentioned previously, septal deviation, hypertrophic turbinates, sinonasal polyps, and other forms of local anatomic obstruction may contribute to chronic rhinitis and are relative indications for surgical intervention due to nasal obstruction.

Surgery is considered in other cases of rhinitis recalcitrant to medical therapy to address specific symptoms in NAR rhinitis and allow topical medications to reach the mucosa. Little debate exists about the consideration of surgery in chronic sinonasal inflammatory disease that is resistant to medical therapy. Tissue conservation and mucosal-sparing techniques are used wherever possible to retain physiologic function and reduce the risk of chronic problems related with surgery, including persistent disease.

In addition to highly vascular mucosa, the membranes of the inferior turbinates contain venous sinusoids surrounded by smooth muscle fibers under autonomic control; there is also a rich supply of mucous and serous glands.[13,56] Hypertrophy that is unresponsive to medical therapy can be addressed in a variety of ways: direct steroid injection; submucosal electrocautery; laser ablation; submucosal resection, including the use of the microdebrider; lateral displacement or outfracture; partial turbinectomy; and radiofrequency ablation. The goals are to use conservative approaches to minimize interference with turbinate function and overall nasal health. Various techniques are also available when contemplating a septoplasty, including submusouc resection and the endoscopic-assisted treatment of the septal deviation.

Vidian neuroectomy is performed to address persistent rhinorrhea resistant to conservative measures. Historically, various approaches have been used: transantral, transpalatal, transethmoid, and transnasal.[57] Current trends favor endoscopic transnasal approaches. This approach has a lower morbidity rate as compared with other methods.[58,59] Complications associated with the procedure include decreased lacrimation, mucosal engorgement when supine, dysesthesia, and recurrence of initial symptoms presumably from re-innervation.

## SUMMARY

It is easy to wield a diagnosis of vasomotor rhinitis on those patients who lack an immunologic response to inhalant allergens and suffer with chronic nasal symptoms. However, NAR can be the result from a myriad of medical issues (eg,

---

**Box 1**
**Summary of nonallergic rhinitis**

*History*
- Medical problems
  - Coexistent sinonasal problems
  - Systemic problems with sinonasal extension
- Medications
- Family history
- Environmental triggers
  - Situations
  - Timing
  - Exacerbating/relieving factors

*Physical examination*
- Full head and neck examination
- Nasal endoscopy
  - Mucosal changes
  - Anatomic findings
  - Presence of a mass lesion

*Diagnostic tests*
- Allergy testing
- Olfactory function testing
- Cytologic examination of nasal secretions
- CT scan if concern for sinus involvement
- Acoustic rhinometry

*Forms of rhinitis*
- NARES
- Hormone-related
- Medication-induced
- Irritant
  - Occupational
- Idiopathic

*Treatment*
- Avoidance
- Medication trials
  - Topical nasal steroids
  - Topical nasal antihistamines
  - Adjunctive medications
    - Nasal anticholinergic sprays
    - Oral antihistamines
- Surgery
  - Anatomic obstruction
  - Turbinate reduction for persistent vascular engorgement
  - Vidian neurectomy

medication usage, hormonal imbalances, systemic medical problems) as well as occupational exposures. Since the facial plastic surgeon often takes a thorough history before performing surgery, she or he will have already gathered much of the information that can point to the diagnosis of NAR. Nasal endoscopy is an important of the examination in evaluating the status of the nasal mucosa and in the recognition of additional problem such as sinonasal polyps or septal deviation.

Patient education is a key factor in managing NAR. Avoidance measures and medical therapy will often take care of the majority of symptomatology and mucosal disease seen in NAR. Sometimes a multidisciplinary approach is required to address the related systemic medical problems. The facial plastic surgeon is aware of the many adjunctive surgical procedures that can be performed at the time of cosmetic or nasal reconstructive surgery. Taking an organized, stepwise approach in addressing the sinonasal symptoms and the underlying problems related to NAR before surgery will aid in positive postoperative outcomes and patient satisfaction (**Box 1**).

## REFERENCES

1. Settipane RA, Lieberman P. Update on nonallergic rhinitis. Ann Allergy Asthma Immunol 2001;86(5): 494–507.
2. Smith TL. Vasomotor rhinitis is not a wastebasket diagnosis. Arch Otolaryngol Head Neck Surg 2003;129(5):584–7.
3. Lund VJ, Preziosi P, Hercberg S, et al. Yearly incidence of rhinitis, nasal bleeding, and other symptoms in mature women. Rhinology 2006;44(1): 26–31.
4. Settipane RA, Charnock DR. Epidemiology of rhinitis: allergic and nonallergic. Clin Allergy Immunol 2007;19:23–4.
5. Ryden O, Andersson B, Andersson M. Disease perception and social behaviour in persistent rhinitis: a comparison between patients with allergic and nonallergic rhinitis. Allergy 2004;59(4):461–4.
6. Levenson T, Greenberger PA. Pathophysiology and therapy for allergic and nonallergic rhinitis: an updated review. Allergy Asthma Proc 1997;18(4): 213–20.
7. AHRQ Publication No. 02–E023: Management of allergic and nonallergic rhinitis, Summary, Evidence Report/Technology Assessment No. 54, May 2002, Agency for Healthcare Research and Quality. Available at: www.ahrq.gov. Accessed September 1, 2003.
8. Fokkens WJ. Thoughts on the pathophysiology of nonallergic rhinitis. Curr Allergy Asthma Rep 2002; 2(3):203–9.
9. The broad spectrum of rhinitis: etiology, diagnosis, and advances in treatment. Presented at the National Allergy Advisory Council Meeting (NAAC)- St Thomas, U.S. Virgin Islands, October 16, 1999.
10. Joe SA, Patel S. Nonallergic rhinitis. In: Flint PW, Haughey BH, Richardson MA, et al, editors. Otolaryngology head and neck surgery. 5th edition. Philadelphia: Mosby Elsevier; 2010. p. 694–702.
11. Corey JP. Vasomotor rhinitis should not be a wastebasket diagnosis. Arch Otolaryngol Head Neck Surg 2003;129:588–9.
12. Sanico A, Togias A. Noninfectious, nonallergic rhinitis (NINAR): considerations on possible mechanisms. Am J Rhinol 1998;12(1):65–72.
13. Spector SL. Allergic and nonallergic rhinitis: update on pathophysiology and clinical management. Am J Ther 1995;2(4):290–5.
14. Powe DG, Jones NS. Local mucosal immunoglobulin E production: does allergy exist in nonallergic rhinitis? Clin Exp Allergy 2006;36(11):1367–72.
15. Rondon C, Romero JJ, Lopez S, et al. Local IgE production and positive nasal provocation test in patients with persistent nonallergic rhinitis. J Allergy Clin Immunol 2007;119(4):899–905.
16. Wedback A, Enbom H, Erisson NE, et al. Seasonal nonallergic rhinitis (SNAR)—a new disease entity? A clinical and immunological comparison between SNAR, seasonal allergic rhinitis and persistent nonallergic rhinitis. Rhinology 2005;43(2): 86–92.
17. Togias AG. Nonallergic rhinitis. In: Mygind N, Naclerio RM, editors. Allergic and nonallergic rhinitis clinical aspects. Munskgaard. Copenhagen (Denmark): WB Saunders; 1993. p. 159–66.
18. Stjarne P, Lundblad L, Anggard A, et al. Local capsaicin treatment of the nasal mucosa reduces symptoms in patients with nonallergic nasal hyperreactivity. Am J Rhinol 1991;5:145.
19. Borum P. Nasal methacholine challenge: a test for the measurement of nasal reactivity. J Allergy Clin Immunol 1979;63(4):253–7.
20. Shahab R, Phillips DE, Jones AS. Prostaglandins, leukotrienes and perennial rhinitis. J Laryngol Otol 2004;118(7):500–7.
21. Hilberg O, Grymer LF, Pedersen OF. Nasal histamine challenge in nonallergic and allergic subjects evaluated by acoustic rhinometry. Allergy 1995;50(2): 166–73.
22. Naclerio RM, Proud D, Kagey-sobotka A, et al. Cold dry air-induced rhinitis: effect of inhalation and exhalation through the nose. J Appl Physiol 1995;79(2): 467–71.

23. Togias A, Proud D, Lawrence M, et al. The osmolality of nasal secretions increases when inflammatory mediators are released in response to inhalation of cold, dry air. Am Rev Respir Dis 1988;137(3):625–9.

24. Togias A, Naclerio RM, Proud D, et al. Studies on the allergic and nonallergic nasal inflammation. J Allergy Clin Immunol 1988;81(5):782–90.

25. Togias A, Naclerio RM. Cold air-induced rhinitis. Clin Allergy Immunol 2007;19:267–81.

26. Togias A, Naclerio RM, Proud D, et al. Mediator release during nasal provocation: a model to investigate the pathophysiology of rhinitis. Am J Med 1985;79(Suppl 6A):26–33.

27. Jacobs RL, Freedman PM, Boswell RN. Nonallergic rhinitis with eosinophilia (NARES syndrome): clinical and immunologic presentation. J Allergy Clin Immunol 1981;67(4):253–62.

28. Amin K, Rinne J, Simola M, et al. Inflammatory cell and epithelial characteristics of perennial allergic and nonallergic rhinitis with a symptom history of 1 to 3 years' duration. J Allergy Clin Immunol 2001; 107(2):249–57.

29. Ellegard E, Hellgren M, Toren K, et al. The incidence of pregnancy rhinitis. Gynecol Obstet Invest 2000; 49(2):98–101.

30. Sobol SE, Frenkiel S, Nachtigal D, et al. Clinical manifestations of sinonasal pathology during pregnancy. J Otolaryngol 2001;30(1):24–8.

31. Georgitis JW. Prevalence and differential diagnosis of chronic rhinitis. Curr Allergy Asthma Rep 2001; 1(3):202–6.

32. Ellegard FK, Karlsson NG, Ellegard LH. Rhinitis in the menstrual cycle, pregnancy, and some endocrine disorders. Clin Allergy Immunol 2007;19:305–21.

33. Togias AG, Naclerio RM, Proud D. Nasal challenge with cold, dry air results in the production of inflammatory mediators: possible mast cell involvement. J Clin Invest 1985;76(4):1375–81.

34. Raphael G, Raphael MH, Kaliner M. Gustatory rhinitis: a syndrome of food-induced rhinorrhea. J Allergy Clin Immunol 1989,83(1):110–5.

35. Baraniuk JN, Kaliner MA. Functional activity of upper-airway nerves. In: Busse W, Holgate S, editors. Asthma and rhinitis. Cambridge (MA): Blackwell Scientific; 1995. p. 652.

36. Bardana EJ. Occupational asthma and related respiratory disorders. Dis Mon 1995;41:143.

37. Meggs WJ. Neurogenic inflammation and sensitivity to environmental chemicals. Environ Health Perspect 1993;101(3):234–8.

38. Hellgren J, Toren K. Nonallergic occupational rhinitis. Clin Allergy Immunol 2007;19:241–8.

39. Puchner TC, Fink JN. Occupational rhinitis. Immunol Allergy Clin North Am 2000;20(2):303–22.

40. Jaradeh SS, Smith TL, Torrico L, et al. Autonomic nervous system: evaluation of patients with vasomotor rhinitis. Laryngoscope 2000;110(11): 1828–31.

41. Staevska MT, Baraniuk JN. Differential diagnosis of persistent nonallergic rhinitis and rhinosinusitis syndromes. Clin Allergy Immunol 2007;19:35–53.

42. Meggs WJ, Cleveland CH Jr. Rhinolaryngoscopic examination of patients with the multiple chemical sensitivity syndrome. Arch Environ Health 1993; 48(1):14–8.

43. Simola M, Malmberg H. Sense of smell in allergic and nonallergic rhinitis. Allergy 1998;53:190–4.

44. Mamikoglu B, Houser SM, Corey JP. An interpretation method for objective assessment of nasal congestion with acoustic rhinometry. Laryngoscope 2002;112(5):926–9.

45. Gosepath J, Amedee RG, Mann WJ. Nasal provocation testing as an international standard for evaluation of allergic and nonallergic rhinitis. Laryngoscope 2005;115(3):512–6.

46. Pipkorn U, Proud D, Lichtenstein LM, et al. Inhibition of mediator release in allergic rhinitis by pretreatment with topical glucocorticosteroids. N Engl J Med 1987;316:1506–10.

47. Webb DR, Meltzer EO, Finn AF, et al. Intranasal fluticasone propionate is effective for perennial nonallergic rhinitis with or without eosinophilia. Ann Allergy Asthma Immunol 2002;88(4):385–90.

48. Highlights of prescribing information. Astra Zeneca Web site. Available at: http://www1.astrazeneca-us. com/pi/Rhinocort_Aqua.pdf. Accessed September 1, 2011.

49. Banov CH, Lieberman PL. Efficacy of azelastine nasal spray in the treatment of vasomotor (perennial nonallergic) rhinitis. Ann Allergy Asthma Immunol 2001;86(1):28–35.

50. Gehanno P, Deschamps E, Garay E, et al. Vasomotor rhinitis: clinical efficacy of azelastine nasal spray in comparison with placebo. ORL J Otorhinolaryngol Relat Spec 2001;63(2):76–81.

51. Lieberman PL, Kaliner MA, Wheeler WJ. Open-labeled evaluations of azelastine nasal spray in patients with seasonal allergic rhinitis and nonallergic vasomotor rhinitis. Curr Med Res Opin 2005;21(4):611–8.

52. Purello-D'Ambrosio F, Isola S, Ricciardi L, et al. A controlled study of the effectiveness of loratadine in combination with flunisolide in the treatment of nonallergic rhinitis with eosinophilia (NARES). Clin Exp Allergy 1999,29(8):1143–7.

53. Greiner AN, Meltzer EO. Pharmacologic rationale for treating allergic and nonallergic rhinitis. J Allergy Clin Immunol 2006;118(5):985–98.

54. Finn AF Jr, Aaronson D, Korenblat P, et al. Ipratropium bromide nasal spray .03% provides additional relief from rhinorrhea when combined with terfenadine in perennial rhinitis patients; a randomized, double-blind, active-controlled trial. Am J Rhinol 1998;12(6):441–9.

55. Grossman J, Banov C, Boggs P, et al. Use of ipratropium bromide nasal spray in chronic treatment of nonallergic perennial rhinitis, alone and in combination with other perennial rhinitis medications. J Allergy Clin Immunol 1995;95:1123–7.

56. Moore GF, Freeman TJ, Ogren FP, et al. Extended follow-up of total inferior turbinate resection for relief of chronic nasal obstruction. Laryngoscope 1985; 95:1095–9.

57. Fernandes CM. Bilateral transnasal vidian neurectomy in the management of chronic rhinitis. J Laryngol Otol 1994;108(7):569–73.

58. Kamel R, Zaher S. Endoscopic transnasal vidian neurectomy. Laryngoscope 1991;101(3):316–9.

59. Liu SC, Wang HW, Su WF. Endoscopic vidian neurectomy: the value of preoperative computed tomographic guidance. Arch Otolaryngol Head Neck Surg 2010;136(6):595–602.

# Allergic Skin Disease

Andrew J. Heller, MD[a,b,*]

## KEYWORDS

- Atopic dermatitis • Contact dermatitis
- Allergic skin disease • Allergy

---

**Key Points:** Allergic Skin Disease

- Atopic dermatitis and contact dermatitis are two very common skin disorders which can be associated with significant patient discomfort and morbidity in the peri-surgical time-frame.
- Skin care, anti-inflammatories, anti-infectives, and anti-pruritics are all vital to the successful treatment and prophylaxis of atopic dermatitis.
- Identification of the causative agent and avoidance are the hallmarks of successful treatment for contact dermatitis.
- Flares of allergic skin disease are common following surgery, but can be minimized through proper prophylaxis individualized to each patient.

---

The skin is the largest immunologic organ in humans, accounting for approximately 15% of our body weight, with a surface area of 1-2 square meters in an adult. Immune dysfunction can affect this massive organ in several ways, with some of the more common being atopic dermatitis, contact dermatitis, urticaria, angioedema, psoriasis, and autoimmune blistering disorders. As surgeons who often violate the skin and mucosa it is vital to understand these disease processes and how they may interact with the expected outcomes of surgical procedures. This review will focus on the two allergic skin diseases which are most common in the world, but the least familiar to Otolaryngologists - atopic dermatitis and contact dermatitis.

## ATOPIC DERMATITIS

Atopic dermatitis, also referred to as eczema, is an extremely prevalent chronic inflammatory skin disease. It affects up to 20% of the pediatric population, making it the most common skin disorder in children. The disease can persist into adulthood, and rarely manifest later in life, affecting 3% to 5% of the adult population. Its prevalence is higher in industrialized nations, and, within these nations, higher in urban than rural regions.[1] In the late 1990s, 2 studies showed the prevalence of atopic dermatitis to be increasing. One involved a questionnaire of Swedish school children (3000 7-year-olds) in both 1979 and 1991. The prevalence of atopic dermatitis more than doubled in that time (7%–18%).[2] A second study examined 7000 Japanese school children, revealing a doubling of the number of affected children aged 9 to 12 years in a 20-year period, and a fivefold prevalence increase in 18-year-olds in the same time period.[3]

Seventy percent of patients with atopic dermatitis develop symptoms before the age of 5 years,

---

The author has nothing to disclose.

[a] Section of Otolaryngology–Head and Neck Surgery, McGuire Veterans Affairs Medical Center, Surgical Service (112), 1201 Broad Rock Boulevard, Richmond, VA 23249, USA
[b] Department of Otolaryngology–Head and Neck Surgery, Virginia, Commonwealth University, Richmond, VA, USA
* Section of Otolaryngology–Head and Neck Surgery, McGuire Veterans Affairs Medical Center, Surgical Service (112), 1201 Broad Rock Boulevard, Richmond, VA 23249.
*E-mail address:* Andrew.Heller@va.gov

Facial Plast Surg Clin N Am 20 (2012) 31–42
doi:10.1016/j.fsc.2011.10.004
1064-7406/12/$ – see front matter Published by Elsevier Inc.

with symptoms frequently present in early infancy. Thirty percent of these patients develop asthma, and 35% develop allergic rhinitis.[4] It has long been debated whether it is the disorder of atopic dermatitis that predisposes to this presumed worsening and extension of allergic disease. This progression of allergic diatheses has been commonly referred to as the atopic march and led to use of antihistamines in young children with atopic dermatitis to try to prevent the development of these other disease processes. There is no evidence to support this approach, except when specific sensitizations to other antigens are identified.[5] There are other factors that may predispose to the development of asthma in these patients, particularly filaggrin defects, which are discussed later.

The natural history of atopic dermatitis leads to resolution of disease by early adolescence in 60% of children, although 50% may recur into adulthood. Predictors of persistent disease include early onset, severe early disease, asthma and allergic rhinitis, and family history. Evidence of food and inhalant allergy before the age of 2 years also predicts severe disease.[6]

The cause of atopic dermatitis remains elusive, although many clues have been gained in recent years. There seems to be a role for genetic predisposition, immune responses, epithelial barrier dysfunction, infectious agents, and environmental factors. With regard to genetics, when both parents have atopic dermatitis, there is an 81% chance that the child will have the disease. When only 1 parent is affected, the child may show signs of eczema 59% of the time.[7] Several suspect genes have been identified, including some coding for components of the immunoglobulin E (IgE) receptor and Th2 cytokines.[8,9] Perhaps most promising are those mutations that seem to interact with the epithelial barrier of the skin.

### The Epithelial Barrier

One of the most important roles performed by the skin is as a barrier between the external environment and our internal milieu. It decreases the permeability to water, allowing decreased evaporation and maintenance of an intact, fluid-filled barrier. It also has antimicrobial and antioxidant effects. Normal skin has an acidic pH, which is inhospitable to colonization by certain bacteria, particularly Staphylococcus aureus. The skin is the body's largest immune organ, serving as a site for the initiation of both cellular and humoral immune reactions. Disorders have been identified in atopic dermatitis that can interfere with any or all of these integumentary functions.[10]

Filaggrin is a protein normally produced in skin. Its name comes from filament of aggregation integrity of the skin. As skin matures, the cells get smaller until they form the dead stratum corneum, which forms the main barrier between the environment and our immune system. Filaggrin is produced in the granular layer. It is initially formed as profilaggrin, which is broken down into filaggrin and some breakdown products. These products include keratohyaline granules and free amino acids that eventually find their way to the stratum corneum and contribute to the acid mantle, preventing bacterial colonization. The filaggrin then binds to, and is responsible for, keratin aggregation. It induces the cytoskeleton to collapse and form corneocytes. The corneocytes are then cross-linked and form a strong barrier to evaporation.[11]

Filaggrin mutations have previously been identified in patients with ichthyosis vulgaris, and, more recently, loss-of-function null mutations have been identified in patients with atopic dermatitis. Filaggrin mutations have been associated with early onset of disease and eczema-associated asthma.[12] This association with asthma takes away from the atopic march hypothesis and explains the airway hyperreactivity in terms of a defect in the epithelial lining of the airway. The importance of filaggrin is further highlighted by a study that showed that patients with atopic dermatitis had low filaggrin expression, even if they did not have full loss-of-function mutations.[13]

A loss of filaggrin function or expression leads to a weakening of the epithelial barrier by decreasing the strength of the stratum corneum. This weakening causes excess water evaporation and drying of the skin. In addition, decreased breakdown of profilaggrin ultimately leads to an alkalinization of the skin surface, making the environment more hospitable to pathologic bacterial colonization.[11]

The alkalinization of the skin has another effect: upregulation of serine proteases. These important enzymes activate proinflammatory cytokines in the skin. They also lead to production of proteins that decrease integrity and cohesion in the skin, as well as downregulating lipid production, which further weakens the permeability barrier. An acquired or inherited increase in the activity of serine protease may be the inciting event in some cases of atopic dermatitis.[14]

Inflammation plays a major role in the pathogenesis of atopic dermatitis. A Th2-predominant reaction is present in acute flares, as shown by the production of interleukin (IL)-13, IL-4, and IL-5. Langerhans cells are hyperactive, overstimulating the T cells. Phosphodiesterase regulation is faulty, causing excessive cytokine production.

There is also a humoral immune response, with increased production of IgE in up to 80% of cases (often caused by staphylococcus toxin superantigens). When a barrier defect is present, cytokine and growth factor production is increased, leading to increased DNA transcription and epidermal hyperplasia, thus accounting for the lichenification that can be seen in many patients with atopic dermatitis. Chemokines are also produced, attracting inflammatory cells and stimulating the production of Th2 cytokines, which has the effect of stimulating further inflammation and decreasing filaggrin production, further damaging the epithelial barrier.[15]

The itch-scratch cycle is often described as the root cause of atopic dermatitis, and it is part of the vicious cycle seen in these patients. An example of this cycle might start with alkalinization of the skin by using the wrong soap. This alkalinization then upregulates the serine proteases, which initiate a cellular inflammatory cascade. This inflammation has several effects, including decreased production of filaggrin, which further weakens the epithelial barrier and water evaporates. Mediators of pruritus are also released, causing the patient to scratch. The scratch and water loss further damage the barrier, and the cycle begins again. The best way to break the itch-scratch cycle is to keep the skin hydrated and decrease the inflammatory response, and this forms the backbone of any treatment plan for atopic dermatitis.

## Clinical Presentation of Atopic Dermatitis

Patients with atopic dermatitis have dry, itchy, flaky skin. There may be oozing, weeping, and fissuring of the skin. Other features include erythema, excoriation, edema, and lichenification. In infants and young children, the facial and extensor surfaces of the skin are most frequently involved. The diaper area is usually spared; this is probably the best example of the benefit of scratch prevention: the diaper area is spared because the infants cannot get under the diaper to scratch. In older children and adults, the flexural surfaces become more involved. Oozing and weeping may signify a secondary bacterial infection. Dennie-Morgan lines, the folds and wrinkles in the infraorbital skin, may be exaggerated, and the same can apply to palmar creases of the hands. There may be pigmentary changes, with actively involved skin being a little darker than uninvolved skin. As it heals, skin that was involved may be lighter because of a decreased change with tanning. Hyperkeratosis pilaris, an accentuation of the hair follicles, is common on the face and upper arms.

Patients with atopic dermatitis experience their disease in different ways, but one thing is universal: pruritus. They can usually tell a flare is coming by the onset of the itch. The initial insult to the skin may not have been noticed. The flares may involve multiple sites or be isolated to 1 region, and patients can flare twice a month or twice per year. Each patient with atopic dermatitis is different and their disease severity must be graded and treated appropriately.

## Management of Atopic Dermatitis

### Skin care
Hydration of the skin is the mainstay of treatment of atopic dermatitis, and simple baths are the first step. Baths have been a controversial subject in the past, with some believing that bathing dries the skin. This statement is true because of the phenomenon of wet evaporation, especially with hot water. However, bathing hydrates the skin; patients should not wait long enough for the water to evaporate. This warning has led to the 3-minute rule, which states that an emollient should be applied to the skin within 3 minutes of exiting the bath.[16]

Baths are recommended for patients with atopic dermatitis, usually daily, with only gentle, nonalkalinizing soaps. Patients should avoid irritating oils and bath salts and never use a scrub brush or wash cloth, which might irritate the skin. After the bath, they should blot dry or drip dry before applying any medication and emollient within 3 minutes.

Emollients are as important as the baths. These patients have a deficiency in the barrier that keeps moisture in the skin, so moisture must be constantly replaced. This moisturizing should be in the form of an ointment or cream. Lotions should be avoided because they tend to have large amounts of water in them that evaporates and can dry the skin. Ointments are helpful for thick, fissured, lichenified skin, but they are aesthetically undesirable because of their greasy appearance. Many use a cream during the day, but an ointment at night, for this reason. There are several gentle emollients on the market.

When a flare is particularly severe, hydration may need to be more aggressive, and wet wraps may be the solution. After the bath, an antiinflammatory medication is applied, followed by an emollient. The affected areas are then covered with soft bandages that are damp. These damp bandages are then covered again by dry ones. Wet wraps not only increase hydration, but increase steroid penetration, serve as a scratch barrier, and allow rapid healing of excoriated lesions.[16]

All skin irritants should be avoided in the patient with atopic dermatitis. These irritants include soaps, detergents, and moisturizers that are alkalinizing. Laundry detergents should be liquid and mild, with an extra rinse cycle to ensure their complete removal from clothing. Heat and perspiration can irritate the skin and sunburn can be devastating. Use of a good sunscreen is a vital part of any atopic dermatitis treatment plan. Physical barriers are better than chemical, so zinc oxide or titanium oxide should be preferred. Occlusive and scratchy clothing should also be avoided. Patients do best with loose-fitting cotton, silk, and cotton blends.

### Antiinflammatory medication

After hydration, the next important step in the treatment of atopic dermatitis is stopping the inflammation, and this is most often accomplished through the use of topical corticosteroids. Topical corticosteroids are safe and effective when used correctly. Possible side effects of topical corticosteroids include atrophy of the skin, telangiectasia development, dyspigmentation, perioral dermatitis, and striae. It is important for the provider to be familiar with the various strengths of topical corticosteroids available. Low-strength preparations (eg, hydrocortisone) are not effective for moderate to severe disease, and it would not be prudent to prescribe an ultra–high-dose formulation (eg, clobetasol) to treat the face where skin thinning and telangiectasias are a concern. Ointments generally have a higher potency than creams. Fluticasone propionate and mometasone furoate are the only preparations that have proven efficacy against atopic dermatitis in daily dosing. The ointment formulations of these are considered high potency, whereas the creams are midpotency.[17]

An alternative for topical antiinflammatory treatment in these patients is a calcineurin inhibitor, which are nonsteroidal topical immunomodulators, and the 2 available preparations are tacrolimus and pimecrolimus. When a T cell is presented with an antigen, calcium production is increased, causing calcineurin and calmodulin to bind intracellularly, ultimately leading to increased Th1 cytokine production.

By blocking calcineurin, these medications decrease cytokine production and block the inflammatory cascade. They have proved to be efficacious in mild to moderate atopic dermatitis.[18]

The advantage of topical calcineurin inhibitors is that they are steroid sparing and do not have the typical side effects associated with topical corticosteroids. They are safe to use on the face and the thin skinfolds of the body. There may be a transient burning or stinging with the initial applications, but they are typically well tolerated. The US Food and Drug Administration (FDA) has placed a black-box warning on these agents because of an increased lymphoma risk in animal studies, and perhaps in humans on systemic doses. There is no scientific evidence to support an increased risk of malignancy caused by topical treatment with calcineurin inhibitors.[19] These agents continue to be used routinely, but are reserved for second-line therapy, as recommended by the FDA.

### Secondary infection

S aureus colonization is common in atopic dermatitis, with infections becoming evident in up to 80% of patients. Involved skin starts crusting, with pustules consistent with impetigo and folliculitis. Inflammatory cells are then activated, which leads to increased pruritus, scratching, and initiation of the whole vicious cycle, which continues to exacerbate and spread not only the atopic dermatitis flare but the infection as well. In addition, the staphylococcus toxins serve as superantigens, activating the immune system nonspecifically and greatly increasing the production of IgE. Up to 80% of the increased IgE in patients with atopic dermatitis is directed at the staphylococcus exotoxin.[20]

Treatment of acute infection usually involves parenteral antibiotics. Topical antibiotics can be used, but those preparations often contain preservatives and other substances that can exacerbate atopic dermatitis, or even cause a contact dermatitis. The most commonly used antibiotics are cefadroxil, cephalexin, cefdinir, trimethoprim/sulfa, and tetracycline.[21] Bleach baths are also effective in both active skin infection and prevention of colonization. Bleach is sodium hypochlorite, which has broad antimicrobial activity because of its action of oxidizing bacteria. There is no known resistance and it is nontoxic to human skin at dilute concentrations, similar to a chlorinated swimming pool. One-eighth to one-quarter of a cup of bleach is added to a full tub of water, and a typical bath is taken, lasting approximately 10 minutes. Twice-weekly bleach baths may decrease the likelihood of acute infection. One study has shown a significant decrease in the severity of atopic dermatitis when twice-weekly bleach baths are combined with intranasal mupirocin.[22]

Other infections can be devastating to the patient with atopic dermatitis and must be in the differential any time a change to the typical appearance of affected skin is identified.[23] Eczema herpeticum is characterized by ulcerative lesions caused by the herpes virus. A Tzanck smear can confirm the diagnosis and treatment is with parenteral acyclovir.

Tinea infections have an advancing border, with central clearing. A KOH prep can confirm the diagnosis and treatment involves antifungals. Molluscum contagiosum can also complicate atopic dermatitis. This condition is characterized by papules with central vesiculation. Treatment is difficult, because most of the typical antiwart medications can exacerbate the skin disease.

### Allergy role in atopic dermatitis

Allergy has long been suspected to play a role in atopic dermatitis, and it seems that food allergy can be a major contributor to the disease. Up to 37% of children less than 5 years of age with moderate to severe atopic dermatitis have IgE-mediated food allergy.[24] It is still unclear whether exposure to certain suspect foods can exacerbate disease. Several studies have endeavored to show improvement in atopic dermatitis when avoidance of identified allergenic foods is practiced, but there is little evidence to support the hypothesis.[25] Some studies did show a significant decrease in pruritus when patients allergic to egg practiced strict avoidance.[26–28] When foods are removed from the diet and tolerance develops, it seems they can be safely returned to the diet without exacerbation of skin disease.[29] When standard treatment of atopic dermatitis fails to lead to improvement, testing and treatment of food allergies should be considered. Ninety percent of the positive food reactions in these patients are to 1 or more of 6 foods:

1. Egg
2. Nut
3. Milk
4. Soy
5. Wheat
6. Fish.

Sensitization to aeroallergens may be seen in patients with atopic dermatitis, although there does not seem to be a significantly higher prevalence than in the general population. However, aeroallergens can exacerbate atopic dermatitis either through inhalation or direct contact. The most important allergens involved are dust mite, animal dander, and pollens. The role of dust mite is supported by patch tests, avoidance studies, and high IgE titers to mite antigens in a large proportion of patients with atopic dermatitis.[30] The positive effect of house dust mite avoidance has been shown in several studies.[31] A work-up for inhalant allergy should only be performed in patients with atopic dermatitis if the history otherwise suggests aeroallergen sensitization. Patch testing to common aeroallergens, especially dust mite, should be considered in refractory cases.

### Pruritus

Controlling the pruritus is the most difficult aspect of treatment of atopic dermatitis. If patients can stop scratching, the epithelial barrier has time to heal and recovery is much quicker and complete. Scratching also promotes secondary infection. The best tools for pruritus at this time are the first-generation antihistamines. These medications are not good at stopping the itch, but the sedative qualities are effective. Preparations chosen for this task are typically diphenhydramine, hydroxyzine, or doxepine, but they need to be used in higher doses than are typically seen for allergic rhinitis. Driving should not be allowed while taking these medications at these dosages. There are some topical preparations available for itch relief, the most popular being pramoxine for patients with atopic dermatitis. Topical diphenhydramine and doxepine should be avoided in these patients because they are strong sensitizers. Second-generation, nonsedating antihistamines seem to have little or no value in treating these patients.[32]

### Systemic therapy for atopic dermatitis

Phototherapy and photochemotherapy have been used for several decades in patients with difficult-to-treat atopic dermatitis. It has been repeatedly shown to significantly induce therapeutic beneficial effects at a low cost. Currently, it is most often used as part of a rotational treatment regimen to avoid long-term adverse effects of other medications.[33]

There are systemic options available for atopic dermatitis, but they should be reserved for difficult cases in which all of the treatment recommendations discussed earlier have failed. Systemic corticosteroids should only be used in crisis situations. They work well to treat a severe acute flare, but their use is also associated with a strong rebound effect, often leaving the patient with worse disease than when they began. Other systemic immunomodulators have been used with some success, including cyclosporine A, mycophenolate mofetil, and azathioprine. Interferon γ, infliximab, efalizumab, and omalizumab have also been used in isolated cases, with some success.[1]

### Proactive treatment of atopic dermatitis

Every patient with atopic dermatitis should have an action plan to outline the proper treatment of their disease, whether all skin is uninvolved, they have a mild flare, or a severe outbreak. The action plan should be based on the general supportive care involving skin hydration and barrier therapy (eg, emollients, baths) along with avoidance of irritants. It should include the topical antiinflammatory to be used in the event of a mild disease flare (perhaps a low-dose steroid such as 2.5% hydrocortisone), as well as the choice for a more severe flare (eg, 0.1% mometasone). When the higher-dose steroid is needed, the plan should include instructions on tapering to a lower-dose topical corticosteroid before discontinuing its use, thereby avoiding a rebound flare.

Treatment between flares has proved to be beneficial for patients with atopic dermatitis. They should always avoid skin irritants and practice good skin hydration, but the addition of an antiinflammatory has proved beneficial as well. One study of 376 patients with moderate to severe atopic dermatitis proved that those treated with a twice-weekly steroid ointment (fluticasone) were 5.8 times less likely to flare than controls.[34] In another study, 383 patients were evaluated for the effectiveness of tacrolimus, used proactively 3 times per week. Patients on tacrolimus maintenance had significantly fewer disease relapse days and more flare-free days than controls.[35]

### Atopic Dermatitis and the Rhinoplasty Patient

Any surgical procedure puts patients with atopic dermatitis at risk for an acute flare of their disease. This risk must be weighed against the potential benefits of the surgery when making a decision to proceed. There have been no controlled studies examining any protocol to prevent disease activation in these patients. The following recommendations are based on the science of the disease process and the known benefits of standard therapy, along with anecdotal reports from physicians who have dealt with this issue in the past.

Patients should be instructed to maximize their routine skin maintenance during the week leading up to the surgery, behaving as if they had a flare. This strategy may include increased use of emollient ointments following daily short baths. Two bleach baths during this week may be beneficial as well. Use of antiinflammatory medication in this setting is controversial, but many recommend 2 applications of a low-dose topical steroid (no stronger on the face) or 3 applications of a calcineurin inhibitor, if this is what the patient has used in the past. Some go so far as to use a daily topical antiinflammatory leading up to the surgery, being cognizant of the potential effects on wound healing.

At the time of surgery, the skin prep must be as gentle as possible. The friction associated with the usual perioperative cleansing is enough to initiate a flare on its own. The antiseptic used should also be carefully selected. Chlorhexidine and betadine may be safe because of their slightly acidic pHs, but betadine usually contains alcohol, which may be more drying. Regardless of which substance is used, it must be applied in a gentle manner, with a nonabrasive sponge. When the surgery is complete, a similar sponge can be used to gently clean the prep area, or it may be left in place for patients to wash away at home with their soap of choice. It would be wise to apply an emollient to the entire surgical field at the end of the case. Antibiotic ointment can be used if the patient has not had problems with them in the past.

Patients should be instructed to continue their increased skin care for 1 more week, along with gentle wound care. A topical steroid or calcineurin inhibitor can also be used in a similar fashion to the week before surgery. If a flare does occur, the patient should be prepared and treat it as they would any other exacerbation of their disease.

## CONTACT DERMATITIS

Contact dermatitis is a common inflammatory skin condition, characterized by erythema and edema occurring after contact with a foreign substance. The 12-month prevalence of occupational contact dermatitis has been shown to be 1700 cases per 10,000 workers.[36] Natural resources and mining, manufacturing, and health services have the highest rates of affected individuals.[37] Contact dermatitis ranks second only to traumatic injury as the most common type of occupational disease.[38] However, the disease is more than an occupational entity. It affects individuals from all walks of life, with sensitizations and reactions to everyday substances causing extreme discomfort and disrupting the quality of life for hundreds of thousands of patients.

It may be categorized as either allergic contact dermatitis, accounting for 20% of cases, or irritant contact dermatitis seen in the other 80%. There are many factors that affect the response in contact dermatitis, but at the heart of the issue are 85,000 chemicals, more than 3700 of which have been identified as contact allergens. Many allergens can serve as irritants and chemical irritants can also produce sensitizing allergic reactions, so differentiating between the 2 types can be difficult.[39]

Contact dermatitis usually manifests as erythema and scaling with well-demarcated borders. In the irritant form of the disease, the skin lesions are often painful, and may be described as burning or stinging. The demarcation in these cases is often sharp. In contrast, the skin lesions in allergic contact dermatitis can be extremely pruritic; the itch is usually the predominant feature. The edges of the skin disruption can be less distinct in these patients. Irritant contact dermatitis is most often seen on the hands, but can occur in other regions (eg, lips with excessive lip licking, diaper area caused by irritant diaper dermatitis). Allergic contact dermatitis can occur anywhere. These 2 forms of disease can also overlap.

Irritant contact dermatitis is a result of skin injury, direct cytotoxic effects, or cutaneous inflammation from direct contact with an irritant. This inflammation is a more recent discovery, involving upregulation and recruitment of chemokine genes, regulated by T-cell effector cytokines. Allergic contact dermatitis is caused by a type IV, delayed hypersensitivity reaction. This reaction requires prior sensitization to the involved substance, and leads to the reaction being delayed by 48 hours.

The diagnosis of contact dermatitis is most often made through history and physical examination. The location of the lesions, combined with a history of exposures in that area in the past few days, can often be enough to lead to an avoidance trial (eg, earlobes from nickel-containing earrings, area of the skin treated with a topical antibiotic). When the diagnosis is in question or the avoidance trial is not successful, patch testing can be performed. Patch testing is the only practical, scientific, and objective method for the diagnosis of allergic contact dermatitis and is discussed further later.

## Testing for Contact Dermatitis

Patch testing involves the application of potential allergenic substances to the surface of the skin, leaving them in place for 48 hours to assess for delayed-type hypersensitivity reactions to the allergens. Ninety percent of allergists currently use a commercially available patch test known as the TRUE test (thin-layered rapid-use epicutaneous test) (Allerderm, Phoenix, AZ, USA). This test consists of 3 self-adhering strips, containing 29 antigens, covering some of the most common causes of allergic contact dermatitis. The strips are applied to the upper back and removed after 48 hours. The first reading is done 30 minutes later. A second reading is required to detect reactions that may be more delayed, and this is done at 72 or 96 hours, or even a week later. Thirty percent of negative tests at 48 hours may be positive on delayed readings. Patients are instructed to report any positive reactions to their provider for up to 3 weeks. Neomycin and corticosteroid reactions may not be apparent until 7 days after application. A reaction that is positive at the immediate reading but negative at 72 hours is likely an irritant, not an allergen.[40]

Allergens not found in the TRUE test panel can frequently cause allergic contact dermatitis. The North American Contact Dermatitis Group has ranked the most common allergens as causative agents for allergic contact dermatitis. This list includes at least 3 substances that are not included in the TRUE panel: gold, bacitracin, and methyl dibromoglutaronitrile (a common component of cosmetics). The North American Contact Dermatitis Group has compiled a series of 65 to 70 antigens that they recommend as an optimal panel for patch testing. Use of this panel would be less likely to miss a cause of allergic contact dermatitis, but is more labor intensive, requiring filling of each individual well with the antigen to be tested.[41]

Standardized test panels are available from several manufacturers. Kits are also available for specific exposure patterns, such as hairdressers, shoes, plants, photoallergens, vehicles, metals, antibiotics, and corticosteroids. When a particular personal hygiene product is suspected, the cosmetic industry may supply blind antigens for testing. However, they will not tell you what they are unless you have a positive result. Personal products can also be applied to the wells in a patch test and tested undiluted or in diluted concentrations.[40]

Patch test results are generally reported as weak positive with erythema, infiltration, and possibly papules; strong positive with erythema, infiltration, papules, and vesicles; or extreme positive with bullae and ulcerations. If a result is marginal, it is prudent to wait until 96 hours. If the intensity and/or pruritus worsen, it is likely allergic. Irritant substances can cause false-positives, again making the delayed reading important. Patch test results can be confirmed or denied through an open application test in which the suspect personal product is applied to the antecubital fossa 2 times per day for 5 to 7 days. Absence of a reaction makes contact dermatitis from this substance unlikely.

## Common Contact Allergens

### Urushiol

One of the most common causes of allergic contact dermatitis, and the easiest to diagnose, is exposure to urushiol, a substance in the sap of *Rhus* plants (poison ivy, oak, and sumac). Rhus plants can brush against the skin, causing linear streaks of erythema and vesicles. This type of contact dermatitis often covers large areas of the body because the urushiol can be spread to other regions, including the face and genitals, by direct contact. More than 70% of people exposed to these plants become sensitized.[42]

## Topical medications

Allergic contact dermatitis to topical medication is common. Neomycin is the most frequently encountered culprit, being the third most common overall contact allergen in North America. Its incidence seems to be increasing and cross-sensitivity is frequently seen with gentamycin, kanamycin, streptomycin, and tobramycin. The only safe topical antibiotic for use in these patients is mupirocin. Neomycin contact dermatitis accounts for more than 10% of shoe-induced dermatitis. The reason seems to relate to the absorption of neomycin into the leather and fabric of shoes. In these cases, an abrasion on the foot treated with neomycin allows the agent to seep into the shoes. When the shoes are worn again a year later, the contactant is still present and a reaction occurs. These shoes must be discarded, but the problem does not arise in all shoe leather.[43]

Topical corticosteroids were voted the 2005 Allergen of the Year by the North American Contact Dermatitis Group. The prevalence of reactions to these agents seems to be increasing, but clinicians may be better at detecting them because of increased awareness, an expanded market, and improved patch testing procedures. Allergic contact dermatitis to corticosteroids should be considered in stasis ulcers and chronic eczema, when dermatitis fails to respond to corticosteroids, and when dermatitis worsens with treatment. There are structural subtypes of corticosteroids based on immune recognition sites, and a reaction to one of these classes does not preclude use of one of the others. For example, hydrocortisone, a class A steroid with a C17 short-chain ester does not cross-react with betamethasone, a class C steroid with a C16 methyl group. Steroids are most often patch tested using tixocortol (class A), budesonide (class B and D), and the patient's own commercial steroid preparation; this accounts for up 91% of corticosteroid allergy.[44] Other panels are available for more extensive testing, if desired.

Topical anesthetics, including benzocaine, tetracaine, and dibucaine, can be causative in allergic contact dermatitis. Thimerosol, a preservative in many topical medications, vaccines, cosmetics, and contact lens solutions, can also be an allergen. Topical quinolones have also been associated with contact dermatitis.[38]

## Rubber

Allergic contact dermatitis to rubber and its components is a complex problem. Mercaptobenzothiazole, thiuram mix, black rubber mix, carba mix, and mercapto mix have all been studied in routine patch testing. Most rubber-sensitive individuals are positive to several of these antigens and cross-sensitization is common.[45] This type of contact allergy is a large component of latex allergy, but does not tell the entire story. There are components of latex that are not available for testing, making the diagnosis more difficult.

## Cosmetics

There are more than 2800 fragrance ingredients in a database maintained by the Research Institute for Fragrance Materials, Inc. One-hundred of these are known allergens. Any given fragrance is a complex substance containing hundreds of different chemicals, and these are the most common cause of allergic contact dermatitis caused by cosmetics. Balsam of Peru and Fragrance Mix" are components of the TRUE test that can diagnose many of these patients. When a fragrance allergen is identified, it is important to educate the patient on the term unscented used in the cosmetic industry. This term erroneously suggests that a product does not contain a fragrance, when a masking fragrance is present. In contrast, fragrance-free products are generally acceptable for the allergic patient. Products that are fragrance free with botanic extracts are not safe for use in this population.[46] Other components of cosmetics can act as allergens as well. These components include the numerous preservatives, vehicles, and additives used by the industry. In the TRUE test, these are tested as quarternium 15, imidazolinyl urea, diazolidinyl urea, formaldehyde, paraben, and wool alcohols. Although this is a good, representative example, many contactants can still be missed, simply because there are so many.[46]

p-Phenylenediamine is the main contact allergen identified in hair products, including dyes and permanents. It is also present in black henna used for tattooing. It is a common source of allergic contact dermatitis in the hair care industry. p-Phenylenediamine does not cause a reaction if it is fully oxidized, which means that patients with this particular allergy cannot apply hair dye, but they can cut the hair of someone who has had their hair dyed previously. Preparations used for hair permanents work by continually leeching from the hair to which it has been applied. For this reason, the same patient should not cut the hair of someone who has had a permanent in the recent past.[47]

## Metals

Nickel was the Contact Allergen of the Year for 2008, according to the North American Contact Dermatitis Group, with an increasing incidence in the United States (10.5% from 1985 to 1990,

18% in 2004). Body piercing is the most common cause, and ear piercing is thought to account for the high sensitivity documented in children. When school-aged girls are patch tested, those with their ears pierced are sensitive to nickel 13% of the time, whereas only 1% of those without pierced ears are sensitive. All metal pins used for ear piercing release nickel in varying amounts, leading several European nations to legislate the amount of nickel allowed in these piercing instruments. Early results show a significant decrease in the prevalence of nickel allergy in young women after the law was instituted.[48]

There is evidence to support a contribution of dietary nickel to vesicular hand eczema, as well as systemic contact dermatitis.[49] A meta-analysis of systemic cases revealed that approximately 1% of patients with nickel allergy have systemic reactions to the nickel content of a normal diet. Ten percent more react if the exposure is in the range of 0.55 AH to 0.89 AH mg, greater than the normal diet, but easily reached if foods with higher nickel content are eaten. These foods include cocoa, lentil, soybean, fig, cashews, and raspberries.[50]

The use of nickel in biomedical devices, especially in joint prostheses and endovascular stents, has led to increased concerns about the safety of these implants in patients with suspected nickel sensitization. Reports of these types of allergy have led to great variability in the management of these cases. There are no large, evidence-based, prospective studies examining this issue. Some surgeons and cardiologists refer any patient, with even the slightest suspicion of contact dermatitis, for patch testing. A positive test result might lead to the selection of a more expensive and less optimal implant. With regard to endovascular stenting, one study examined coronary in-stent restenosis 6 months after stainless steel stent placement and patch tested 2 months after angioplasty. There were 11 positive patch test reactions in 10 of the patients (8%). All 10 patients with a positive patch test reaction to metal (7 nickel, 4 molybdenum) had in-stent restenosis. This restenosis rate was significantly higher than the nonallergic patients. The clinical history was not predictive of a positive patch test.[51] In another prospective study of 174 stented patients, those with in-stent restenosis had a significantly higher prevalence of positive patch tests to metal (nickel and manganese).[52] Currently, the evidence for complications caused by nickel allergy is weak, with rare proven cases reported in the literature. The need for patch testing is controversial and the results are poorly reliable in predicting or confirming an implant reaction. Although a negative test might be reassuring, if a positive test is achieved, the implant must be removed.

Although mostly used in jewelry, gold is also an antiinflammatory medication, is used in the electroplating industry, and is part of many dental appliances. Allergic contact dermatitis from this metal has become common, with 9.5% of 4101 patch-tested individuals having a positive reaction.[53] The most common sites of involvement are the hands, the face, and the eyelids. The involvement of facial and eyelid skin is intriguing, because gold is not often in direct contact with these areas. It seems that titanium dioxide, found in many cosmetics, adsorbs gold released from jewelry, spreading it across the face.[54]

## Treatment

The primary treatment of any contact dermatitis is identification and avoidance of contact with allergens and irritants. Although history and location of the skin lesions are helpful, there is no substitute for patch testing. In a study evaluating the differences between patch-tested and non–patch-tested patients with allergic contact dermatitis, relief of symptoms was achieved an average of 143 days sooner in those who had undergone a patch test.[55] Once the causative agents are identified, the patient should be provided with instructions detailing the potential sources of the antigen and synonyms by which they may be known. Alternatives and substitutions may be available for any particular antigen, and these are available through the Contact Allergen Replacement Database maintained by the American Contact Dermatitis Society. Simple measures include covering nickel-plated objects (eg, snap-on jeans), washing formaldehyde-containing clothes, and using gloves or other barriers when handling certain chemicals. For nickel-sensitive patients, the widely available dimethylglyoxime swab test can be used on any substance to detect the presence of this sensitized metal.

Supportive care should be offered for relief of pruritus. This care may include cold compresses with water or saline, aluminum subacetate (Burrow solution), calamine, and colloidal oatmeal baths. Excessive washing of the involved areas should be avoided and use of good, gentle emollients, as described earlier for atopic dermatitis, should be considered. An oral, first-generation antihistamine may also be useful against the itch, mostly through its sedating effects.

A topical corticosteroid is the first line-treatment of mild to moderate allergic contact dermatitis, but more severe presentations frequently require systemic corticosteroids. Calcineurin inhibitors have been tried for these patients, but their efficacy in contact dermatitis has not been established. There seems to be some benefit in chronic contact dermatitis of the hands and feet, but further investigation seems necessary.[56]

### Contact Dermatitis and Rhinoplasty

A careful history of contactant allergy should be obtained in any patient being considered for surgery. The surgeon should be mindful of any evidence of dermatitis on the face, eyelids, ear lobes, and hands. Often, patients have been living with these chronic rashes for so long that they neglect to mention them or seek intervention. If a dermatitis is identified, further history might help suggest whether it is a contact dermatitis, as opposed to atopic dermatitis, dishydrosis, or even psoriasis. If contact dermatitis is suspected, patch testing is warranted.

In patients with known allergic contact dermatitis, some adjustments may need to be made to the surgical or in-office practice. Topical antibiotics must be carefully selected in patients with contact allergy. Often, the culprit is neomycin, which can cross-react with many other topical preparations. In these cases, mupirocin should be considered. Nickel allergy is not an absolute contraindication to metal implants, but alternatives should be considered. Resins present in adhesives may cause contact dermatitis to tape. In addition, practice caution when suggesting skin products for these patients with possible allergies to some of the fragrances, preservatives, and additives used in their manufacture.

## SUMMARY

Atopic dermatitis and contact dermatitis are extremely prevalent allergic diseases of the skin that can be devastating to the patient, with symptoms including severe pruritus, pain, and cosmetically unappealing inflammation of the skin. Although the disease processes do not affect the outcome of surgery, the procedures may trigger a relapse of disease, severely affecting quality of life and adversely affecting recovery. Through knowledge of the pathophysiology of atopic dermatitis and the potential causative agents in allergic contact dermatitis, the surgeon can avoid exacerbation of preexisting skin inflammation and assist with treatment if a flare does occur.

## REFERENCES

1. Akdis CA, Akdis M, Bieber T, et al. Diagnosis and treatment of atopic dermatitis in children and adults: European Academy of Allergology and Clinical Immunology/American Academy of Allergy, Asthma and Immunology/PRACTALL Consensus Report. J Allergy Clin Immunol 2006;118(1):152–69.
2. Aberg N, Hesselmar B, Aberg B, et al. Increase of asthma, allergic rhinitis and eczema in Swedish schoolchildren between 1979 and 1991. Clin Exp Allergy 1995;25(9):815–9.
3. Sugiura H, Umemoto N, Deguchi H, et al. Prevalence of childhood and adolescent atopic dermatitis in a Japanese population: comparison with the disease frequency examined 20 years ago. Acta Derm Venereol 1998;78(4):293–4.
4. Williams HC. Epidemiology of atopic dermatitis. Clin Exp Dermatol 2000;25(7):522–9.
5. Wahn U. Allergic factors associated with the development of asthma and the influence of cetirizine in a double-blind, randomised, placebo-controlled trial: first results of ETAC. Early Treatment of the Atopic Child. Pediatr Allergy Immunol 1998;9(3):116–24.
6. Lammintausta K, Kalimo K, Raitala R, et al. Prognosis of atopic dermatitis. A prospective study in early adulthood. Int J Dermatol 1991;30(8):563–8.
7. Uehara M, Kimura C. Descendant family history of atopic dermatitis. Acta Derm Venereol 1993;73(1):62–3.
8. Cox HE, Moffatt MF, Faux JA, et al. Association of atopic dermatitis to the beta subunit of the high affinity immunoglobulin E receptor. Br J Dermatol 1998;138(1):182–7.
9. Forrest S, Dunn K, Elliott K, et al. Identifying genes predisposing to atopic eczema. J Allergy Clin Immunol 1999;104(5):1066–70.
10. Elias PM, Hatano Y, Williams ML. Basis for the barrier abnormality in atopic dermatitis: outside-inside-outside pathogenic mechanisms. J Allergy Clin Immunol 2008;121(6):1337–43.
11. O'Regan GM, Irvine AD. The role of filaggrin in the atopic diathesis. Clin Exp Allergy 2010;40(7):965–72.
12. Baurecht H, Irvine AD, Novak N, et al. Toward a major risk factor for atopic eczema: meta-analysis of filaggrin polymorphism data. J Allergy Clin Immunol 2007;120(6):1406–12.
13. Howell MD, Kim BE, Gao P, et al. Cytokine modulation of atopic dermatitis filaggrin skin expression. J Allergy Clin Immunol 2009;124(3 Suppl 2):R7–12.
14. Hachem JP, Man MQ, Crumrine D, et al. Sustained serine proteases activity by prolonged increase in pH leads to degradation of lipid processing enzymes and profound alterations of barrier function and stratum corneum integrity. J Invest Dermatol 2005;125(3):510–20.
15. Bieber T. Atopic dermatitis. N Engl J Med 2008;358(14):1483–94.
16. Hanifin JM, Cooper KD, Ho VC, et al. Guidelines of care for atopic dermatitis, developed in accordance with the American Academy of Dermatology (AAD)/American Academy of Dermatology Association

"Administrative Regulations for Evidence-Based Clinical Practice Guidelines". J Am Acad Dermatol 2004;50(3):391–404.

17. Boguniewicz M, Eichenfield LF, Hultsch T. Current management of atopic dermatitis and interruption of the atopic march. J Allergy Clin Immunol 2003;112(Suppl 6):S140–50.

18. El-Batawy MM, Bosseila MA, Mashaly HM, et al. Topical calcineurin inhibitors in atopic dermatitis: a systematic review and meta-analysis. J Dermatol Sci 2009;54(2):76–87.

19. Thaci D, Salgo R. Malignancy concerns of topical calcineurin inhibitors for atopic dermatitis: facts and controversies. Clin Dermatol 2010;28(1):52–6.

20. Macias ES, Pereira FA, Rietkerk W, et al. Superantigens in dermatology. J Am Acad Dermatol 2011;64(3):455–72 [quiz: 473–4].

21. Bath-Hextall FJ, Birnie AJ, Ravenscroft JC, et al. Interventions to reduce Staphylococcus aureus in the management of atopic eczema: an updated Cochrane review. Br J Dermatol 2010;163(1):12–26.

22. Huang JT, Abrams M, Tlougan B, et al. Treatment of Staphylococcus aureus colonization in atopic dermatitis decreases disease severity. Pediatrics 2009;123(5):e808–14.

23. Lipozencic J, Wolf R. Atopic dermatitis: an update and review of the literature. Dermatol Clin 2007;25(4):605–12, x.

24. Eigenmann PA, Sicherer SH, Borkowski TA, et al. Prevalence of IgE-mediated food allergy among children with atopic dermatitis. Pediatrics 1998;101(3):E8.

25. Bath-Hextall F, Delamere FM, Williams HC. Dietary exclusions for improving established atopic eczema in adults and children: systematic review. Allergy 2009;64(2):258–64.

26. Atherton DJ, Sewell M, Soothill JF, et al. A double-blind controlled crossover trial of an antigen-avoidance diet in atopic eczema. Lancet 1978;1(8061):401–3.

27. Agata H, Kondo N, Fukutomi O, et al. Effect of elimination diets on food-specific IgE antibodies and lymphocyte proliferative responses to food antigens in atopic dermatitis patients exhibiting sensitivity to food allergens. J Allergy Clin Immunol 1993;91(2):668–79.

28. Lever R, MacDonald C, Waugh P, et al. Randomised controlled trial of advice on an egg exclusion diet in young children with atopic eczema and sensitivity to eggs. Pediatr Allergy Immunol 1998;9(1):13–9.

29. NIAID-Sponsored Expert Panel, Boyce JA, Assa'ad A, et al. Guidelines for the diagnosis and management of food allergy in the United States: report of the NIAID-sponsored expert panel. J Allergy Clin Immunol 2010;126(Suppl 6):S1–58.

30. Platts-Mills TA, Vervloet D, Thomas WR, et al. Indoor allergens and asthma: report of the Third International Workshop. J Allergy Clin Immunol 1997;100(6 Pt 1):S2–24.

31. Tan BB, Weald D, Strickland I, et al. Double-blind controlled trial of effect of housedust-mite allergen avoidance on atopic dermatitis. Lancet 1996;347(8993):15–8.

32. Wahlgren CF, Hagermark O, Bergstrom R. The antipruritic effect of a sedative and a non-sedative antihistamine in atopic dermatitis. Br J Dermatol 1990;122(4):545–51.

33. Byun HJ, Lee HI, Kim B, et al. Full-spectrum light phototherapy for atopic dermatitis. Int J Dermatol 2011;50(1):94–101.

34. Berth-Jones J, Damstra RJ, Golsch S, et al. Twice weekly fluticasone propionate added to emollient maintenance treatment to reduce risk of relapse in atopic dermatitis: randomised, double blind, parallel group study. BMJ 2003;326(7403):1367.

35. Breneman D, Fleischer AB Jr, Abramovits W, et al. Intermittent therapy for flare prevention and long-term disease control in stabilized atopic dermatitis: a randomized comparison of 3-times-weekly applications of tacrolimus ointment versus vehicle. J Am Acad Dermatol 2008;58(6):990–9.

36. Behrens V, Seligman P, Cameron L, et al. The prevalence of back pain, hand discomfort, and dermatitis in the US working population. Am J Public Health 1994;84(11):1780–5.

37. Workplace injuries and illnesses. Washington, DC: US Department of Labor; 2009 (05/2011).

38. American Academy of Allergy Asthma and Immunology, American College of Allergy Asthma and Immunology. Contact dermatitis: a practice parameter. Ann Allergy Asthma Immunol 2006;97(3 Suppl 2):S1–38.

39. Marks J, Elsner P, Deleo V. Contact and occupational dermatology. St Louis (MO): Mosby; 2002.

40. Fonacier LS, Dreskin SC, Leung DY. Allergic skin diseases. J Allergy Clin Immunol 2010;125(2 Suppl 2):S138–49.

41. Zug KA, Warshaw EM, Fowler JF Jr, et al. Patch-test results of the North American Contact Dermatitis Group 2005-2006. Dermatitis 2009;20(3):149–60.

42. Wolf K, Johnson RA, editors. Fitzpatrick's color atlas and synopsis of clinical dermatology. New York: McGraw-Hill; 2009.

43. Gehrig KA, Warshaw EM. Allergic contact dermatitis to topical antibiotics: epidemiology, responsible allergens, and management. J Am Acad Dermatol 2008;58(1):1–21.

44. Bjarnason B, Flosadottir E, Fischer T. Assessment of budesonide patch tests. Contact Dermatitis 1999;41(4):211–7.

45. Bendewald MJ, Farmer SA, Davis MD. An 8-year retrospective review of patch testing with rubber allergens: the Mayo Clinic experience. Dermatitis 2010;21(1):33–40.

46. Castanedo-Tardan MP, Zug KA. Patterns of cosmetic contact allergy. Dermatol Clin 2009;27(3): 265–80, vi.

47. O'Connell RL, White IR, Mc Fadden JP, et al. Hairdressers with dermatitis should always be patch tested regardless of atopy status. Contact Dermatitis 2010;62(3):177–81.

48. Schram SE, Warshaw EM, Laumann A. Nickel hypersensitivity: a clinical review and call to action. Int J Dermatol 2010;49(2):115–25.

49. Kornik R, Zug KA. Nickel. Dermatitis 2008;19(1):3–8.

50. Jensen CS, Menne T, Johansen JD. Systemic contact dermatitis after oral exposure to nickel: a review with a modified meta-analysis. Contact Dermatitis 2006;54(2):79–86.

51. Koster R, Vieluf D, Kiehn M, et al. Nickel and molybdenum contact allergies in patients with coronary in-stent restenosis. Lancet 2000;356 (9245):1895–7.

52. Iijima R, Ikari Y, Amiya E, et al. The impact of metallic allergy on stent implantation: metal allergy and recurrence of in-stent restenosis. Int J Cardiol 2005;104(3):319–25.

53. Fowler J Jr, Taylor J, Storrs F, et al. Gold allergy in North America. Am J Contact Dermat 2001;12(1):3–5.

54. Ehrlich A, Belsito DV. Allergic contact dermatitis to gold. Cutis 2000;65(5):323–6.

55. Rajagopalan R, Kallal JE, Fowler JF Jr, et al. A retrospective evaluation of patch testing in patients diagnosed with allergic contact dermatitis. Cutis 1996;57(5):360–4.

56. Wollina U. The role of topical calcineurin inhibitors for skin diseases other than atopic dermatitis. Am J Clin Dermatol 2007;8(3):157–73.

# Concurrent Rhinoplasty and Endoscopic Sinus Surgery: A Review of the Pros and Cons and a Template for Success

Douglas D. Reh, MD[a],*, Jason Y.K. Chan, MBBS[a],
Patrick J. Byrne, MD[b]

## KEYWORDS

- Endoscopic • Sinus surgery • Rhinoplasty
- Septorhinoplasty • Septoplasty • Sinusitis
- Facial plastic surgery • Concurrent

---

### Key Points

- The performance of concurrent functional endoscopic sinus surgery (FESS) and rhinoplasty is relatively safe and the complication rates are similar to those when the procedures are performed independently.

- Many patients with functional or aesthetic nasal issues who present with nasal obstruction may also have concurrent sinonasal inflammatory disease. A thorough evaluation is required to identify any inflammatory issues such as allergic rhinitis or chronic rhinosinusitis (CRS).

- A comprehensive plan for patients with nasal obstruction must include both surgical and medical treatments including FESS, rhinoplasty, and antiinflammatory medications.

- Surgery for these patients should be performed in a careful, stepwise approach to address the nasal septum, inferior turbinates, paranasal sinuses, and external nasal structures. Careful attention is given to the internal and external nasal valves during rhinoplasty.

---

Since its introduction in 1986 FESS has emerged as the standard surgical treatment of chronic sinusitis.[1] Simultaneously, there has been an increased demand for facial plastic surgery, with many patients interested in improving facial aesthetics as well as their functional nasal issues. During this period, the importance of the nasal valve to functional nasal surgery outcomes has become more apparent. Effective reconstruction of the nasal valves, both internal and external, is critical to optimizing functional outcomes and quality of life.[2] Many of these rhinoplasty candidates have inflammatory rhinitis and CRS that contributes to their nasal breathing difficulties. These issues can be overlooked and failure to address them can lead to inadequate treatment of the patient's sinonasal complaints.

Historically, surgeons were wary of combining sinus surgery and rhinoplasty because of concerns of significant disruption of internal and

Conflict of Interest: None.
Financial Disclosures: None.
[a] Department of Otolaryngology–Head and Neck Surgery, Johns Hopkins Medical Institutions, 601 North Caroline Street, 6th Floor 6240, Baltimore, MD 21287, USA
[b] Division of Facial Plastic and Reconstructive Surgery, Departments of Otolaryngology–Head and Neck Surgery and Dermatology, Johns Hopkins Medical Institutions, Baltimore, MA, USA
* Corresponding author.
E-mail address: dreh1@jhmi.edu

Facial Plast Surg Clin N Am 20 (2012) 43–54
doi:10.1016/j.fsc.2011.10.005

external nasal structures as well as spread of infection to adjacent surgical sites. However, with the advent of minimally invasive techniques for performing FESS there is minimal disruption to nasal structures that support the external nose, and with present perioperative antibiotic therapy, contamination of the external nose from sinusitis is low.[3–5]

## THE PROS AND CONS OF CONCURRENT FESS AND RHINOPLASTY

When considering whether to perform a concurrent FESS and rhinoplasty, the surgeon must weigh the potential risks and benefits of this type of procedure. Fakhri and Citardi[6] describe several potential considerations that argue against the simultaneous performance of these surgical procedures. Millman and Smith[7] describe a case of glabellar abscess, septic shock, and myocarditis after a FESS and rhinoplasty. Fakhri and Citardi[6] suggest that FESS on patients with CRS who are frequently infected may induce bacteremia and that performing osteotomies may allow for a periosteal breach of infection that could result in soft tissue infections. The use of allogenic or synthetic grafts may also increase risks of local infection. Postoperative bleeding and hemorrhage is an inherent risk to both rhinoplasty and FESS. Theoretically this risk may be additive when both procedures are performed at the same time. The potential sites of bleeding differ for each of these procedures and therefore the source of postoperative hemorrhage may be difficult to ascertain.[6]

Rhinoplasty causes intranasal as well as soft tissue postoperative edema, resulting in nasal and periorbital swelling. This edema could conceivably mask a postoperative orbital complication caused by a concurrent FESS.[6] In addition, this situation may make postoperative debridement, which is critical to successful endoscopic sinus surgery (ESS) to reduce crusting and scar formation, difficult. Postoperative debridement requires endoscopic manipulation of the nose and sinonasal passages in the immediate postoperative period. This exercise could cause movement or disruption of the grafts and osteotomies created during the rhinoplasty, leading to a worse aesthetic result. Friedman reported medial collapse of the ascending process of the maxilla after a combined FESS/rhinoplasty, causing collapse of the nasal valve and concavity of the nasal side wall.[8]

Increased risk of soft tissue and nasal infection remains a primary concern when performing concurrent FESS and rhinoplasty. Table 1 outlines

several recent studies that describe concurrent FESS/rhinoplasty. Many of the studies did not report intranasal or soft tissue infections, whereas those studies that did report this complication had a rate of 2% to 2.3%. This finding is consistent with the rates of postoperative rhinoplasty infections, typically reported at between 1.7% and 2.7%.[9–11] Lee and colleagues[12] reported a slightly higher postoperative infection rate, with 4 of their 55 (6%) patients developing cellulitis. Of their cases, 51% were patients who had gross sinonasal purulence evident at the time of surgery, indicating active or acute infection. This situation may have contributed to their higher reported incidence of cellulitis after FESS/rhinoplasty, although none of these patients had gross purulence at the time of surgery. Overall, the rate of postoperative infections in these studies is consistent with those published for FESS and rhinoplasty performed independently. This finding argues against the theory that performing the 2 procedures simultaneously increases the rates of postoperative sinusitis, vestibulitis, or cellulitis.

Three of the concurrent FESS/rhinoplasty studies in **Table 1** reported postoperative epistaxis or hemorrhage, with a rate between 0% and 6.6% across all studies. Postoperative synechiae were also reported in these studies at rates between 4.4% and 22%. Minor complications such as epistaxis, synechiae, and periorbital ecchymosis or emphysema after FESS are reported at rates between 2% and 21%.[13] Minor complications of rhinoplasty such as epistaxis have been reported at rates between 2% and 4%.[14–19] These rates are comparable with those reported in the studies in **Table 1**, which indicates that there is no additive risk of minor complications when performing concurrent FESS and rhinoplasty. The investigators of these studies advocate combining these procedures only in patients with less severe sinus disease arbitrarily assessed by Lund-Mackay scores less than 8.[3,4]

Displacement of nasal structure and grafts caused by endoscopic manipulation as well as inability to perform necessary postoperative FESS debridements secondary to increased intranasal edema has also been discussed as potential contraindications to performing concurrent FESS/rhinoplasty.[6] Although Friedman[8] described a case of posterior prolapse of the ascending process of the maxilla after simultaneous FESS and rhinoplasty, none of the larger case series has reported this problem. Of the studies outlined in **Table 1**, only Sclafeni and Schaefer[3] clearly describe their postoperative debridement regimen. They performed endoscopic debridement

**Table 1**
**Summary of previous concurrent FESS/rhinoplasty studies**

| Study (n) | Procedures | FESS Indication | Complications (n, %) |
|---|---|---|---|
| Sclafani and Schaefer[3] (13) | FESS (n) Closed rhinoplasty (3) Open rhinoplasty (10) | CT evidence of persistent sinusitis after medical therapy | None reported |
| Costa et al[36] (13) | Maxillary/mandibular osteotomies FESS Open rhinoplasty | Endoscopic or CT evidence of anatomic obstruction or inflammatory disease | None reported |
| Inanli et al[37] (45) | FESS Open rhinoplasty | Endoscopic or CT evidence of anatomic obstruction or inflammatory disease[a] | Postoperative hemorrhage (3, 6.6) Synechiae (2, 4.4) Periorbital emphysema (1, 2.2) |
| Kirchner and Dutton[4] (48) | FESS Closed rhinoplasty (27) Open rhinoplasty (21) | Endoscopic or CT evidence of persistent sinusitis after medical therapy | Facial pain (1, 2) Unilateral nasal obstruction (1, 2) Unilateral facial cellulitis (1, 2) |
| Marcus et al[38] (44) | FESS Closed rhinoplasty (27) Open rhinoplasty (17) | Endoscopic or CT evidence of anatomic obstruction or inflammatory disease | Vestibulitis (1, 2.3) Cellulitis (1, 2.3) |
| Lee et al[12] (55) | FESS Open rhinoplasty | Evidence of persistent sinusitis after medical therapy[b] | Postoperative epistaxis (2, 3.6) Cellulitis (4, 6) |
| Toffel[34] (122) | FESS Closed rhinoplasty | Endoscopic or CT evidence of persistent sinusitis after medical therapy | Postoperative hemorrhage (3, 2.5) Synechiae (27, 22) Lamina papyracea defect (2, 1.6) |

[a] Excluded patients with frontal or sphenoid sinusitis.
[b] 51% of cases had acute purulent debris at time of surgery.

at 5 to 7 days after surgery and had their patients start nasal rinses at that time. None of the studies report difficulty with performing sinus debridements or disruption of grafts or osteotomies as a result of endoscopic manipulation in the postoperative period. Sclafeni and Schaefer[3] did find an increased duration of nasal tip and dorsum edema after concurrent FESS and rhinoplasty. These investigators found that the duration of postoperative nasal edema was highly correlated with the severity of sinusitis on patient preoperative computed tomography (CT) scan reflected by their Lund-Mackay scores. The investigators theorize that increased intranasal edema after FESS may cause a secondary impairment in external nasal lymphatic drainage as well as venous congestion.

The aforementioned studies have shown that concomitant FESS and rhinoplasty can be performed safely and effectively. There are several advantages of concurrent FESS and rhinoplasty, many of which stem from the efficiencies gained from performing each procedure simultaneously. The most obvious advantage is that the patient's functional and aesthetic nasal issues can be addressed along with their sinuses in a single, minimally invasive outpatient procedure. Because the patient with CRS and functional nasal issues undergoes 1 definitive procedure, hospital time, surgical costs, and recovery time are reduced. Many patients who present with complex functional and inflammatory issues require a comprehensive evaluation and treatment plan. This goal is most effectively accomplished with a multidisciplinary approach and a medical and surgical treatment plan that efficiently addresses these issues. This approach is described in the following section.

## EVALUATION AND SURGICAL PLANNING FOR THE RHINOPLASTY PATIENT WITH ALLERGIC RHINITIS OR CHRONIC SINUSITIS

Although it has never been prospectively evaluated, many patients with functional or aesthetic nasal issues who present for consideration of rhinoplasty may also have concurrent sinonasal inflammatory disease. Both allergic rhinitis and CRS can cause symptoms of obstructed nasal breathing and congestion. Although both should be treated medically, patients with CRS may also benefit from FESS to improve their symptoms and quality of life. It is important for the physician to be able to distinguish these 2 entities and establish a diagnosis and effective treatment plan before rhinoplasty to optimize the patient's outcome. The surgeon should be able to determine those patients who would benefit from concurrent FESS and rhinoplasty.

Evidence based clinical practice guidelines have been published to assist physicians with the diagnosis and treatment of sinusitis.[20] Three cardinal symptoms have been identified for diagnosing sinusitis based on their high sensitivity and specificity for acute sinusitis.[20] These are purulent nasal discharge, nasal obstruction, and facial pressure, pain, or fullness. Hyposmia is also sensitive for CRS. CRS is defined as the presence of two or more of these symptoms lasting for longer than 12 weeks. Symptom based criteria alone are nonspecific and therefore objective findings of inflammation either on CT scan or endoscopy is required to make the diagnosis.[20] Acute bacterial rhinosinusitis (ABRS) is treated medically and defined as the presence of the three cardinal symptoms and/or signs of inflammation for longer than 10 days or worsening within 10 days.[20] Recurrent acute sinusitis is diagnosed when 4 or more episodes of ABRS occur per year, without signs or symptoms of sinusitis between episodes.[20] Patients with recurrent acute bacterial sinusitis (ABRS) or CRS as defined by the clinical guidelines outlined by Rosenfeld and colleagues who have failed medical therapy are candidates for FESS. Those patients with suspected CRS or recurrent sinusitis who are candidates for rhinoplasty should be evaluated and treated before scheduling them for concurrent FESS/rhinoplasty. The patient's past medical history should include a detailed evaluation of symptoms and their associated time course to ensure that they meet the aforementioned criteria for CRS or recurrent sinusitis. Sinus CT scans should be obtained and nasal endoscopy performed to document the presence of inflammation. For those patients with recurrent sinusitis, a CT scan and endoscopy can be performed to confirm the presence of inflammation during an episode. This strategy is helpful to make an accurate diagnosis and rule out imitators of sinusitis such as headache or migraine disorders, which can manifest with similar symptoms. Although CT scans are not advocated for the diagnosis of ABRS,[20] they may be helpful as a preoperative assessment in patients with recurrent sinusitis to determine which sinuses should be addressed during FESS.

CT scans can also be helpful to identify structural anomalies that can contribute to functional nasal obstruction. **Fig. 1** shows the CT scan of a patient with bilateral nasal obstruction. Her nasal examination showed only mild bilateral internal nasal valve collapse and a subtle septal deviation. However, her CT scan, obtained by the facial plastic surgeon, showed bilateral concha bullosa. Failure to address these issues would have led to inadequate surgical treatment of her nasal symptoms. **Fig. 2** shows the CT scan of a patient who was evaluated with left nasal obstruction greater than right. His nasal examination showed a significant left deviated septum. In addition his CT scan revealed a hyperpneumatized right-sided anterior ethmoid cell that was medializing his right middle turbinate and pushing on the septum. This cell was reduced at the time of his septoplasty to allow for lateralization of the middle turbinate and medialization of his septum. These cases illustrate how CT scans can show anatomic sinonasal abnormalities that should be addressed at the time of septorhinoplasty to maximize surgical outcome.

Similar to allergic rhinitis and nonallergic rhinitis, patients with CRS should be treated with medical

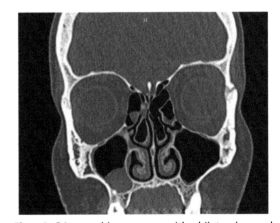

**Fig. 1.** 34-year-old woman with bilateral nasal congestion. On examination she had only mild nasal valve collapse and septal deviation. CT scan revealed bilateral conchal bullosa. Endoscopic reduction was performed bilaterally and she noted significant improvement in her postoperative nasal breathing.

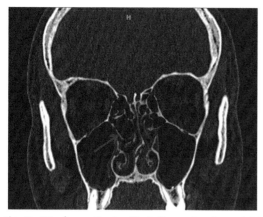

**Fig. 2.** CT of a patient with left greater than right nasal obstruction. On examination he had left nasal septal deviation. His CT revealed hyperpneumatized right anterior ethmoid cell (*arrow*) causing deviation of the ipsilateral middle turbinate and septum. This cell was reduced endoscopically to allow for lateralization of the middle turbinate and straightening of the nasal septum.

Cottle maneuver supporting the upper lateral cartilage should be performed, with any subjective improvement in nasal airflow noted. Identification of the presence of internal or external nasal valve collapse helps the surgeon to determine if using batten grafts to address the internal or external nasal valves, or spreader grafts to address the internal nasal valve is of most benefit to the patient.[24,25]

We advocate a multidisciplinary approach to the evaluation of patients with a history of aesthetic, functional, and inflammatory sinonasal problems. Because these patients often present to a subspecialized otolaryngologist, it is important for the evaluating surgeon to focus on all potential causes of the patient's concerns, even if their treatment is outside the surgeon's surgical expertise. Careful screening is conducted by our facial plastic surgeon (PB) and rhinologist/endoscopic sinus surgeon (DR) during the evaluation of a patient with sinonasal issues. Rhinoplasty candidates with symptoms suggestive of inflammatory sinonasal disease (**Box 1**; **Table 2**) are referred to our

therapy before considering FESS or any surgical procedure. Although there is no consensus on what constitutes maximal medical therapy,[21] generally a 2-week to 4-week treatment regimen with appropriate antibiotics and oral corticosteroids is recommended.[22] For those patients whose symptoms and signs of inflammation persist despite medical therapy, FESS is an effective treatment.[23]

Evaluation of nasal valve disease begins with questions regarding any preferred side of breathing, worsening of breathing under physical strain, improvement on pulling 1 side of the cheek (the instinctive Cottle maneuver), or worsening with certain positions while asleep. During physical examination the surgeon must carefully examine both the external and internal nasal valves. The external nasal valve is the area of the nasal vestibule under the nasal ala formed by the caudal septum, the alar rim, and the medial crura of the alar cartilages. This area represents the first component of nasal resistance. Any caudal septal deviation, concavity of the alar rim, or dynamic functional collapse should be noted. Furthermore, a modified Cottle maneuver is performed using an ear curette to support the lower lateral cartilage in order to determine if there is subjective improvement in nasal obstruction. Next, the internal nasal valve is examined. This area comprises the dorsal septum, the caudal border of the upper lateral cartilage, and the anterior aspect of the inferior turbinate. Any high septal deviation that can compress the internal nasal valve should be noted. The upper lateral cartilage should be examined for concavity or static collapse, and a modified

| Box 1 |
|---|
| **Symptoms associated with allergic and nonallergic rhinitis** |
| *Allergic Rhinitis* |
| Sneezing |
| Itchy eyes/eye rubbing |
| Itchy nose |
| Clear rhinorrhea |
| Seasonal symptoms |
| Family history of allergic rhinitis |
| Eczema or food allergy |
| *Nonallergic Rhinitis* |
| Persistent congestion/rhinorrhea without sneeze or itchy nose |
| Poor response to oral antihistamine |
| Symptoms exacerbated by: |
|     Weather changes |
|     Temperature changes/extremes |
|     Perfumes/odors |
|     Smoke/fumes |
| Older age at onset |
| Absence of allergens as a trigger |
| *Data from* Carr WW, Nelson MR, Hadley JA. Managing rhinitis: strategies for improved patient outcomes. Allergy Asthma Proc 2008;29(4):350. |

**Table 2**
**Definitions for diagnosis of chronic sinusitis and recurrent acute sinusitis**

|  | Definition |
|---|---|
| CRS | 12 wk or longer of 2 or more of the following signs and symptoms:<br>• Mucopurulent drainage<br>• Nasal obstruction (congestion)<br>• Facial pain/pressure/fullness<br>• Reduced sense of smell<br>• And inflammation is documented by 1 or more of the following findings:<br>• Purulent mucus or edema in the middle meatus or ethmoid region<br>• Polyps in nasal cavity or the middle meatus<br>• Radiographic evidence of inflammation of the paranasal sinuses |
| Recurrent acute rhinosinusitis | 4 or more episodes/year of ABRS without signs or symptoms of rhinosinusitis between episodes:<br>• Symptoms of purulent nasal discharge accompanied by nasal obstruction, facial pain/pressure/fullness, or both<br>• Symptoms of acute rhinosinusitis are present 10 d or more beyond the onset of upper respiratory symptoms, or<br>• Symptoms or signs of acute rhinosinusitis worsen within 10 d after an initial improvement (double worsening) |

*Reproduced from* Rosenfeld RM, Andes D, Bhattacharyya N, et al. Clinical practice guideline on adult sinusitis. Otolaryngol Head Neck Surg 2007;137(3):S18; with permission.

endoscopic sinus surgeon for further evaluation, medical treatment, and consideration of FESS. Similarly, patients with sinusitis with functional breathing issues and external structural abnormalities such as internal nasal valve collapse or a twisted nasal dorsum are referred to our facial plastic surgeon. This type of collaboration leads to a comprehensive treatment plan with medical and surgical therapy to optimize outcome and patient satisfaction. These patients often require long-term follow-up and treatment by a rhinologist for their inflammatory sinus disease even after successful FESS. **Fig. 3** outlines a multidisciplinary algorithm for the preoperative evaluation and treatment of patients presenting with aesthetic, functional, and inflammatory sinonasal complaints.

## SURGICAL TECHNIQUE OF CONCURRENT RHINOPLASTY AND FESS

Concurrent rhinoplasty/FESS is scheduled for those patients who require functional and aesthetic rhinoplasty, meet the diagnostic criteria for CRS or recurrent sinusitis, and have failed to improve on medical therapy. Preoperative CT scans are obtained for most patients for the reasons discussed earlier. Patients are evaluated endoscopically 1 to 2 weeks before surgery to ensure they do not have active infection. Although the studies in **Table 1** have shown that there is no

substantially increased risk of a spread of infection from the sinuses to adjacent soft tissue structures during simultaneous rhinoplasty/FESS, we advocate avoiding this procedure on patients with active infection. Those patients who show mucopurulence during the preoperative evaluation are treated with antibiotics before surgery. Surgery is delayed if the infection persists despite antibiotic therapy. In some cases, culture-directed antibiotics are used or FESS is performed without rhinoplasty if the infection cannot be eradicated.

Establishing a consistent surgical sequence is important for successful concurrent rhinoplasty/FESS. It is our experience that rhinoplasty, especially when it involves lateral osteotomies, causes significant intranasal edema that can make FESS difficult and in some cases impossible. We advocate an approach that is consistently outlined in previous studies.[3,4] A septoplasty is performed initially for several reasons. First, this procedure maximizes endoscopic visualization and access to the nasal cavity for performance of the FESS. The septoplasty is usually performed by our endoscopic sinus surgeon (DR) and so it is performed endoscopically. This procedure allows for excellent visualization of posterior deviations and spurs that can obstruct nasal breathing. Cartilage is also harvested from the septum during septoplasty to be used during rhinoplasty by the plastic surgeon (PB) for grafts and struts. The submucoperiosteal flaps are

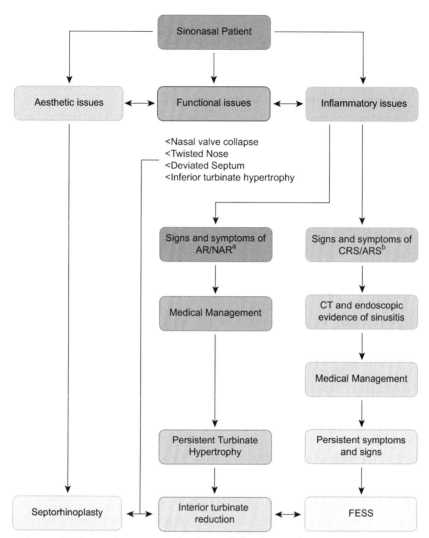

**Fig. 3.** Preoperative evaluation and treatment algorithm of the sinonasal patient. [a] Box 1 documents the signs and symptoms of allergic rhinitis (AR) and nonallergic rhinitis (NAR). [b] Table 2 documents the signs and symptoms of CRS and acute recurrent sinusitis (ARS).

closed at the end of the case, which allows for further manipulation of the septum if needed during the rhinoplasty.

FESS is performed after adequate topical decongestion and injections. Directed maxillary antrostomies, ethmoidectomies, sphenoidotomies, and frontal sinusotomies are completed based on the patient's preoperative assessment, including CT scan, endoscopic evaluation, and symptom history. Inferior turbinoplasty is also performed with either radiofrequency coblation (ArthoCare ENT, Austin, TX, USA) or submucosal microdebridement (Medtronic, Minneapolis, MN, USA). The inferior turbinates are also outfractured, which is an important step toward increasing the nasal cavity volume.

The rhinoplasty maneuvers are chosen based on whether the patient is being treated for nasal valve disease, aesthetic concerns, or both. Particular emphasis is placed on the treatment of the internal, and occasionally external nasal valves. Optimizing the nasal valve anatomy and competency leads to improved functional outcomes.[26]

The key to success begins with effective communication with the endoscopic sinus surgeon. When the endoscopic septoplasty is performed, it is important that the harvested septal cartilage is structurally intact, and of sufficient dimensions to accomplish the required grafting. If this goal is not accomplished, which is particularly common in revision cases, then plans are

**Technique summary from Johns Hopkins: rhinoplasty and FESS**

Septoplasty

- A septoplasty is performed initially to maximize endoscopic visualization and access to the nasal cavity for performance of FESS.
- The septoplasty is usually performed endoscopically, allowing for excellent visualization of posterior deviations and spurs that can obstruct nasal breathing.
- Cartilage is harvested from the septum during septoplasty to be used during rhinoplasty by the plastic surgeon for grafts and struts.
- The submucoperiosteal flaps are closed at the end of the case, allowing for further manipulation of the septum if needed during the rhinoplasty.

FESS

- FESS is performed after adequate topical decongestion and injections.
- Directed maxillary antrostomies, ethmoidectomies, sphenoidotomies, and frontal sinusotomies are completed based on the patient's preoperative assessment.
- Inferior turbinoplasty is also performed with either radiofrequency coblation or submucosal microdebridement
- The inferior turbinates are outfractured, helping increase the nasal cavity volume.

Rhinoplasty

- The key to success begins with effective communication with the endoscopic sinus surgeon.
- When the endoscopic septoplasty is performed, it is important that the harvested septal cartilage is structurally intact, and of sufficient dimensions to accomplish the required grafting.
- If this goal is not accomplished, particularly common in revision cases, then plans are made to harvest additional autologous cartilage. Ear or rib cartilage is used in these situations.
- Rhinoplasty maneuvers are chosen based on whether the patient is being treated for nasal valve disease, aesthetic concerns, or both.
- Emphasis is placed on the treatment of the internal and, occasionally, external nasal valves.
- Optimizing the nasal valve anatomy and competency leads to improved functional outcomes.
- Functional structural integrity is sought for both the static dimensions of the airway (this may require spreader grafts, lateralizing osteotomies, or both), as well as the dynamic lateral nasal sidewall support (which often requires batten grafts, rim grafts, or both).
- Notes are made to precisely diagnose the areas of airway restriction, whether static, dynamic, or both.
- In most functional cases, the placement of any necessary grafts and osteotomies is performed in an endonasal fashion.
- Aesthetic rhinoplasty maneuvers are more likely to require an open approach to afford unsurpassed exposure to optimize accuracy and control.
- The structural approach includes the anatomic dissection and performance of key maneuvers such as the dorsal hump reduction. This procedure is typically performed after elevation of the nasal septal mucosa to allow separation of the upper lateral cartilages from the dorsal septum before hump reduction. This strategy helps to prevent mucosal disruption and the risk of scarring of the internal nasal valve. Spreader grafts are routinely placed after hump reduction to prevent valve collapse (and for asserting control over midvault width, an aesthetic priority).
- The nasal tip work is performed in conjunction with maneuvers to stabilize the nasal base. This work may require columellar strut grafts, septocolumellar sutures, or caudal septal extension grafts.
- We avoid nasal packing in the postoperative period because it reduces patient discomfort after surgery. Although nasal packing can also be used as a splint to hold struts and grafts placed during rhinoplasty, patient discomfort is also associated with these packs, and accidental lateralization of the middle turbinate may occur. If nasal packing is required we recommend that it be placed endoscopically to ensure that the middle turbinates are not lateralized as a result of the packs.
- The middle turbinate can be sutured to the septum during closure of the mucoperiosteal flaps to ensure medialization.
- External thermoplastic splints are placed to stabilize the external nasal structure and nasal bones after rhinoplasty.

made to harvest additional autologous cartilage. Ear or rib cartilage is used in these situations.

The authors advocate a structural approach to both functional and aesthetic rhinoplasty. Functional structural integrity is sought for the static dimensions of the airway (this may require spreader grafts, lateralizing osteotomies, or both) as well as the dynamic lateral nasal sidewall support (which often requires batten grafts, rim grafts, or both). The preoperative history and physical examination are essential toward determining the optimal surgical plan. Notes are made to precisely diagnose the areas of airway restriction, whether static, dynamic, or both. In most functional cases, the placement of any necessary grafts and osteotomies are performed in an endonasal fashion.

Aesthetic rhinoplasty maneuvers are more likely to require an open approach. An open rhinoplasty may be performed after the endoscopic septoplasty with graft harvesting. There are situations, however, in which it is best to perform the septoplasty via an open rhinoplasty approach. Examples include when there is a marked caudal septal deflection or a twisted midvault. These cases require extensive dissection and reconstruction of the septum, occasionally via extracorporeal modifications, and is best performed open. This approach affords unsurpassed exposure to optimize accuracy and control. Keys to the structural approach include the anatomic dissection and performance of key maneuvers such as the dorsal hump reduction. This procedure is typically performed after elevation of the nasal septal mucosa to allow separation of the upper lateral cartilages from the dorsal septum before hump reduction. This strategy helps to prevent mucosal disruption and the risk of scarring of the internal nasal valve. Spreader grafts are routinely placed after hump reduction to prevent valve collapse (and for asserting control over midvault width, an aesthetic priority).

The nasal tip work is performed in conjunction with maneuvers to stabilize the nasal base. This work may require columellar strut grafts, septocolumellar sutures, or caudal septal extension grafts. We have not noticed a significant difference in the healing of the skin soft tissue envelope in aesthetic cases that undergo concurrent FESS.

The early postoperative edema may be somewhat increased however, nasal packs are typically used after FESS and rhinoplasty to control epistaxis and prevent or reduce middle meatal adhesions that can impair sinus drainage postoperatively. Packs are also used to hold grafts and struts positioned during rhinoplasty in place immediately after surgery. The drawback of nasal packing is that there is associated discomfort during the postoperative

period, especially with removal of the packs.[27] Although multiple studies have shown some benefit in terms of controlling epistaxis and reducing middle meatal adhesions, there is no consistent evidence that middle meatal packing improves these outcomes over avoidance of packing.[28] We avoid nasal packing in the postoperative period because it reduces patient discomfort after surgery. The middle turbinate can be sutured to the septum during closure of the mucoperiosteal flaps to ensure medialization.[29] Although nasal packing can also be used as a splint to hold struts and grafts placed during rhinoplasty, patient discomfort is also associated with these packs, and accidental lateralization of the middle turbinate may occur (**Fig. 4**). If nasal packing is required we recommend that it be placed endoscopically to ensure that the middle turbinates are not lateralized as a result of the packs. External thermoplastic splints are placed to stabilize the external nasal structure and nasal bones after rhinoplasty. **Fig. 5** shows endoscopic pictures depicting improvement in nasal cavity volume after concurrent FESS/rhinoplasty.

## POSTOPERATIVE MANAGEMENT AFTER CONCURRENT ESS AND RHINOPLASTY

Perioperative oral corticosteroids have been shown to improve postoperative inflammation.[30] We treat patients after FESS with oral dexamethasone for 1

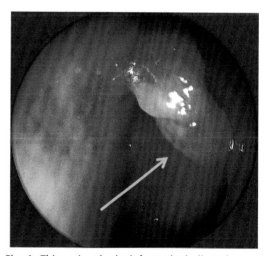

**Fig. 4.** This patient had a left concha bullosa that was reduced endoscopically and bilateral maxillary antrostomies for recurrent maxillary sinusitis. She also underwent bilateral internal nasal valve reconstruction and placement of spreader grafts. Anterior nasal packs were placed to position the grafts during the immediate postoperative period. Postoperative endoscopic examination during debridement revealed lateralization of the concha bullosa with folding of the turbinate (*arrow*) caused by medially placed nasal packs.

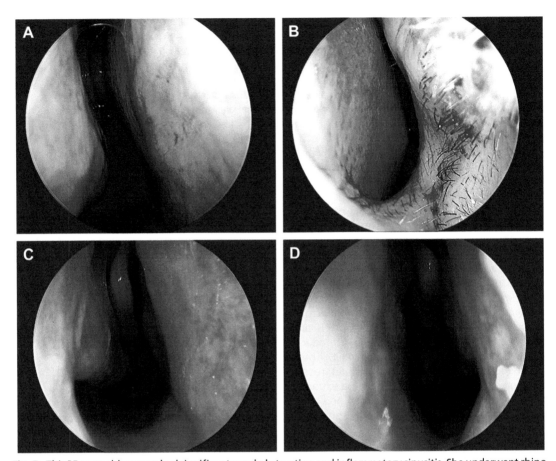

**Fig. 5.** This 35-year-old woman had significant nasal obstruction and inflammatory sinusitis. She underwent rhinoplasty including placement of spreader grafts and repair of internal nasal valve stenosis as well as an endoscopic septoplasty. Bilateral endoscopic maxillary antrostomies and inferior turbinate coblation with outfracture were also performed. (*A*) Preoperative endoscopic view of right nasal cavity showing high septal deflection with obscuring of middle turbinate. (*B*) Preoperative endoscopic picture of extreme left caudal septal deflection with nasal valve collapse. (*C* and *D*) Right and left postoperative endoscopic views, respectively, with significant improvement in nasal cavity volume. The patient noted significant improvement in her nasal breathing postoperatively.

to 2 weeks after surgery. Sinonasal irrigations are started on postoperative day 1 to help eliminate blood clots and crusting that can impair healing. Similar to Sclafeni and Schaefer,[3] post-FESS endoscopic debridement after adequate topical decongestion and anesthetic is performed at 1 week. At that time any nasal splints are also removed. Care is used to avoid significant manipulation of the external nasal structures with the endoscope during the debridement. If further debridement is required this is performed 2 to 3 weeks after surgery. Previous studies that attempted to determine the benefit of postoperative antibiotic after FESS are contradictory.[31,32] Studies that investigated postoperative antibiotics after rhinoplasty have found no benefit compared with intraoperative or preoperative antibiotics alone.[10,33] There are no prospective studies that have determined the

specific benefit of postoperative antibiotic for simultaneous FESS/rhinoplasty. Studies that describe concurrent FESS/rhinoplasty advocate treating with intraoperative as well as postoperative antibiotics for 5 to 10 days.[3,34] Topical nasal steroids are started at 4 weeks after surgery for patients with a significant history of inflammatory disease. These steroids have been shown to be effective in treating long-term symptoms.[35]

## SUMMARY

Historically concurrent FESS/rhinoplasty was avoided because of concerns of increased risk of complications, especially postoperative soft tissue infections and disruption of nasal structures caused by manipulation during endoscopic procedures. Recent studies have shown that

FESS/rhinoplasty can be performed simultaneously with good outcomes and no significant increase in complications. A thorough and effective approach to the patient with sinonasal obstruction requires attention to aesthetic, functional, and inflammatory issues. Medical treatment is an important adjuvant to surgery to optimize outcomes by improving patient symptoms longterm. Surgery for these patients should be performed in a careful, stepwise approach to address the nasal septum, inferior turbinates, paranasal sinuses, and external nasal structures.

## REFERENCES

1. Kennedy DW. Functional endoscopic sinus surgery. Technique. Arch Otolaryngol 1985;111(10):643–9.
2. Most SP. Analysis of outcomes after functional rhinoplasty using a disease-specific quality-of-life instrument. Arch Facial Plast Surg 2006;8(5):306–9.
3. Sclafani AP, Schaefer SD. Triological thesis: concurrent endoscopic sinus surgery and cosmetic rhinoplasty: rationale, risks, rewards, and reality. Laryngoscope 2009;119(4):778–91.
4. Kircher ML, Dutton JM. Concurrent endoscopic sinus surgery and rhinoplasty. Am J Rhinol 2006;20(5):485–8.
5. McGraw-Wall B, MacGregor AR. Concurrent functional endoscopic sinus surgery and rhinoplasty: pros. Facial Plast Surg Clin N Am 2004;12(4):425–49, vi.
6. Fakhri S, Citardi MJ. Considerations against concurrent functional endoscopic sinus surgery and rhinoplasty. Facial Plast Surg Clin N Am 2004;12(4):431–4, vi.
7. Millman B, Smith R. The potential pitfalls of concurrent rhinoplasty and endoscopic sinus surgery. Laryngoscope 2002;112(7 Pt 1):1193–6.
8. Friedman WH. Endorhinoplasty. Simultaneous rhinoplasty and endoscopic ethmoidectomy. Facial Plast Surg Clin N Am 1999;7:357–71.
9. Pirsig W, Schafer J. The importance of antibiotic treatment in functional and aesthetic rhinosurgery. Rhinol Suppl 1988;4:3–11.
10. Andrews PJ, East CA, Jayaraj SM, et al. Prophylactic vs postoperative antibiotic use in complex septorhinoplasty surgery: a prospective, randomized, single-blind trial comparing efficacy. Arch Facial Plast Surg 2006;8(2):84–7.
11. Klabunde EH, Falces E. Incidence of complications in cosmetic rhinoplasties. Plast Reconstr Surg 1964;34:192–6.
12. Lee JH, Sherris DA, Moore EJ. Combined open septorhinoplasty and functional endoscopic sinus surgery. Otolaryngol Head Neck Surg 2005;133(3):436–40.
13. Kinsella JB, Calhoun KH, Bradfield JJ, et al. Complications of endoscopic sinus surgery in a residency training program. Laryngoscope 1995;105(10):1029–32.
14. Holt GR, Garner ET, McLarey D. Postoperative sequelae and complications of rhinoplasty. Otolaryngol Clin N Am 1987;20(4):853–76.
15. Carr WW, Nelson MR, Hadley JA. Managing rhinitis: strategies for improved patient outcomes. Allergy Asthma Proc 2008;29(4):349–57.
16. Nassef M, Shapiro G, Casale TB. Identifying and managing rhinitis and its subtypes: allergic and nonallergic components–a consensus report and materials from the Respiratory and Allergic Disease Foundation. Curr Med Res Opin 2006;22(12):2541–8.
17. Benninger M, Farrar JR, Blaiss M, et al. Evaluating approved medications to treat allergic rhinitis in the United States: an evidence-based review of efficacy for nasal symptoms by class. Ann Allergy Asthma Immunol 2010;104(1):13–29.
18. Bhandarkar ND, Smith TL. Outcomes of surgery for inferior turbinate hypertrophy. Curr Opin Otolaryngol Head Neck Surg 2010;18(1):49–53.
19. Lethbridge-Cejku M, Schiller JS, Bernadel L. Summary health statistics for U.S. adults: National Health Interview Survey, 2002. Vital Health Stat 10 2004;(222):1–151.
20. Rosenfeld RM, Andes D, Bhattacharyya N, et al. Clinical practice guideline on adult sinusitis. Otolaryngol Head Neck Surg 2007;137(3):S1–31.
21. Dubin MG, Liu C, Lin SY, et al. American Rhinologic Society member survey on "maximal medical therapy" for chronic rhinosinusitis. Am J Rhinol 2007;21(4):483–8.
22. Lund VJ. Maximal medical therapy for chronic rhinosinusitis. Otolaryngol Clin N Am 2005;38(6):1301–10, x.
23. Smith TL, Litvack JR, Hwang PH, et al. Determinants of outcomes of sinus surgery: a multi-institutional prospective cohort study. Otolaryngol Head Neck Surg 2010;142(1):55–63.
24. Fischer H, Gubisch W. Nasal valves–importance and surgical procedures. Facial Plast Surg 2006;22(4):266–80.
25. Constantinides M, Galli SK, Miller PJ. A simple and reliable method of patient evaluation in the surgical treatment of nasal obstruction. Ear Nose Throat J 2002;81(10):734–7.
26. Rhee JS, Arganbright JM, McMullin BT, et al. Evidence supporting functional rhinoplasty or nasal valve repair: a 25-year systematic review. Otolaryngol Head Neck Surg 2008;139(1):10–20.
27. Mo JH, Han DH, Shin HW, et al. No packing versus packing after endoscopic sinus surgery: pursuit of patients' comfort after surgery. Am J Rhinol 2008;22(5):525–8.
28. Weitzel EK, Wormald PJ. A scientific review of middle meatal packing/stents. Am J Rhinol 2008;22(3):302–7.
29. Hewitt KM, Orlandi RR. Suture medialization of the middle turbinates during endoscopic sinus surgery. Ear Nose Throat J 2008;87(12):E11.

30. Wright ED, Agrawal S. Impact of perioperative systemic steroids on surgical outcomes in patients with chronic rhinosinusitis with polyposis: evaluation with the novel Perioperative Sinus Endoscopy (POSE) scoring system. Laryngoscope 2007; 117(11 Pt 2 Suppl 115):1–28.

31. Albu S, Gocea A, Mitre I. Preoperative treatment with topical corticoids and bleeding during primary endoscopic sinus surgery. Otolaryngol Head Neck Surg 2010;143(4):573–8.

32. Jiang RS, Liang KL, Yang KY, et al. Postoperative antibiotic care after functional endoscopic sinus surgery. Am J Rhinol 2008;22(6):608–12.

33. Rajan GP, Fergie N, Fischer U, et al. Antibiotic prophylaxis in septorhinoplasty? A prospective, randomized study. Plast Reconstr Surg 2005;116(7): 1995–8.

34. Toffel PH. Simultaneous secure endoscopic sinus surgery and rhinoplasty. Ear Nose Throat J 1994; 73(8):554–6, 558–60, 565.

35. Joe SA, Thambi R, Huang J. A systematic review of the use of intranasal steroids in the treatment of chronic rhinosinusitis. Otolaryngol Head Neck Surg 2008;139(3):340–7.

36. Costa F, Robiony M, Salvo I, et al. Simultaneous functional endoscopic sinus surgery and esthetic rhinoplasty in orthognathic patients. J Oral Maxillofac Surg 2008;66(7):1370–7.

37. Inanli S, Sari M, Yazici MZ. The results of concurrent functional endoscopic sinus surgery and rhinoplasty. J Craniofac Surg 2008;19(3):701–4.

38. Marcus B, Patel Z, Busquets J, et al. The utility of concurrent rhinoplasty and sinus surgery: a 2-team approach. Arch Facial Plast Surg 2006;8(4):260–2.

# The Unified Airway

John H. Krouse, MD, PhD

## KEYWORDS

- Airway • Respiratory tract • Pathophysiology
- Cardiopulmonary risk

---

### Key Points

- The upper and lower airways function as an integrated, interdependent respiratory unit, known as the unified airway.
- Stimuli that affect one portion of the airway often trigger concurrent pathophysiologic changes at sites distant from the initial stimulus.
- Asthma coexists with allergic and nonallergic rhinitis in 40% of individuals, and with chronic rhinosinusitis in up to 50% of individuals.
- Recognition of increased prevalence of lower airway disease among patients with rhinitis and rhinosinusitis is important in the perioperative management of patients undergoing nasal surgery.
- Patients with significant upper airway symptoms should be screened by history for the presence of cough and exercise-induced wheezing and dyspnea.
- Nasal packing should be used judiciously in elderly patients and those with underlying cardiopulmonary diseases because of increased risk of hypoxia and arrhythmia.
- An appreciation of the unified airway among facial plastic surgeons permits safer nasal surgery.

---

Within the specialty of otolaryngology, as well as in related fields of respiratory medicine (allergy/immunology, pulmonary medicine), there has been growing appreciation for the integrated function of the upper and lower respiratory systems in health and disease. Recognition of shared physiologic mechanisms and epidemiologic links between various respiratory disorders has promoted development of a conceptual model of integrated respiratory function known as the unified airway. This interdependence of the upper and lower respiratory systems has been described in a growing number of papers in the past 2 decades, permitting a better understanding of these shared mechanisms, as well as suggesting a more comprehensive approach to diseases such as asthma, rhinitis, and rhinosinusitis.[1]

In the unified airway model, the entire respiratory system, from the middle ear to the distal bronchioles, functions in an integrated, interdependent manner, and can be conceptualized as an organized unit. A variety of mechanisms seem to be involved in driving this unified respiratory system, but the most important seems to be shared inflammation as a result of continual communication among cellular and humoral components of the immune system.[2,3] Inflammation that is initiated in one discrete portion of the respiratory tract can be propagated and sustained through locoregional and systemic processes, with resulting effects at a site distant from the original locus of inflammation.[4] In addition, the implication is that exacerbations of ongoing disease in one portion of the respiratory system lead to concurrent or subsequent worsening of disease in other respiratory units.

In the past decade, a major advance in the recognition of unified airway disease was noted

---

Department of Otolaryngology–Head and Neck Surgery, Temple University School of Medicine, 3440 North Broad Street, Kresge West #300, Philadelphia, PA 19140, USA
*E-mail address:* jkrouse@temple.edu

Facial Plast Surg Clin N Am 20 (2012) 55–60
doi:10.1016/j.fsc.2011.10.006
1064-7406/12/$ – see front matter © 2012 Elsevier Inc. All rights reserved.

with the development of the ARIA (Allergic Rhinitis and its Impact on Asthma) guidelines. First published in 2002,[5] and then revised in 2010,[6] ARIA presents a comprehensive review of international data and expert opinion that describes the intimate relationship between components of the respiratory tract. The ARIA panel emphasizes interdependence within the respiratory system, as well as detailing the expanding database supporting these relationships. Of note for the rhinoplasty surgeon is ARIA's recommendation that "when considering a diagnosis of rhinitis or asthma, an evaluation of both the upper and lower airways should be made."[5] The implication of this statement is that caution should be taken when considering cosmetic nasal surgery in patients with asthma, not only because of their potentially increased risk from anesthesia, but because active rhinitis is common among patients with asthma.

This article first examines the epidemiologic and pathophysiologic relationships that exist among inflammatory diseases of the respiratory system, including issues that affect the nasal airway in allergic and nonallergic rhinitis and in chronic rhinosinusitis. It specifically looks at some potential issues that may be important in considering rhinoplasty among patients with unified airway disease.

## EPIDEMIOLOGIC RELATIONSHIPS

The relationship between allergic rhinitis and asthma has been appreciated for many years. It is known that, among patients diagnosed with allergic rhinitis, the likelihood of developing asthma during a 20-year period is 3 times greater among allergic individuals than in their nonallergic counterparts.[7,8] In addition, about one-third of patients with rhinitis have concurrent asthma at the time of their rhinitis diagnosis, whereas more than 80% of patients with asthma have active rhinitis, either allergic or nonallergic.[9] Furthermore, the presence of rhinitis not only predicts the concurrence of clinically significant asthma but also is associated with the degree of bronchial hyperreactivity among patients not yet diagnosed with asthma.[10] There seems to be an ongoing persistent inflammation in patients with allergic rhinitis and asthma, even in the absence of currently active disease.

In addition, there is a consistent relationship noted among patients with asthma and those with chronic rhinosinusitis (CRS). Although the prevalence of asthma in the general community is estimated at about 7%, among patients with CRS, the prevalence increases to about 20%.[11] The prevalence continues to increase to 42% among patients with CRS undergoing sinus surgery, and,

among patients with CRS with polyps and those with asthma, to a prevalence of more than 50%.[12] Successful medical and surgical treatment of CRS is associated with improvement in patient symptoms and quality of life, as well as improved level of asthma control.[13] Not only is surgery thought to improve nasal respiration among patients with CRS, but to decrease the load of immunoactive tissue, with subsequent reduction in propagation of inflammation to the lower airways.

## PATHOPHYSIOLOGIC MECHANISMS AND CLINICAL AIRWAY DISEASE

Pathophysiologic mechanisms that are involved in rhinitis, CRS, and asthma are similar and interrelated. Two areas are important to consider among patients being considered for rhinoplasty surgery:

1. Impairment in nasal respiration
2. Shared inflammation.

Sufficient nasal respiration is thought to be vital physiologically in sustaining maximal pulmonary function, especially among patients with bronchial hyperreactivity and asthma. In a classic study, when patients with asthma were allowed to breathe either with their noses obstructed or open, obstruction of the nose was associated with a decline in pulmonary function and worsening bronchospasm when these patients increased their exercise activity.[14] Nasal obstruction inhibits the conditioning of inspired air by the nasal turbinates, and seems to contribute to lower respiratory symptoms and the development of asthma.[15] With the increase in ventilatory rate during exercise, greater volumes of cold dry air with higher amounts of particulate matter are delivered to the lungs; interference with nasal breathing, as with nasal obstruction, inhibit the nose's ability to filter and condition inspired air, contributing to lower airway inflammation and bronchospasm.[16]

The effect of nasal obstruction on the mechanics of breathing and lower airway resistance was extensively studied by Ogura and colleagues[17,18] in the 1960s, who noted that total nasal obstruction increases pulmonary resistance, and postulated a reflex mechanism controlling bronchial smooth muscle physiology. This effect of nasal obstruction on increased pulmonary resistance and bronchoconstriction has also been noted with the use of packs placed during nasal surgery.[19] There is increased risk for these effects on pulmonary physiology among patients with asthma, who have decreased pulmonary reserve, increased bronchial hyperreactivity, and increased epithelial inflammation.

In addition to the adverse effects of nasal obstruction on lower airway mechanics and function, there is a prominent role for shared inflammatory processes across both the upper and lower respiratory systems. The inflammatory cascade in the airway is initiated in allergic patients with deposition of allergen on the mucosa, usually first in the nose. Both early-phase and late-phase responses are then initiated in susceptible individuals. Allergic responses involve the degranulation of mast cells on cross-linking of adjacent immunoglobulin-E (IgE) molecules, resulting in the release of histamine and other inflammatory mediators into the local tissues. Other stimulatory and regulatory responses are also initiated, including the recruitment of T-helper 2 (Th2) cells, as well as late-phase mediators, especially eosinophils, proinflammatory cytokines, and leukotrienes, sustaining the allergic response and promoting persistent inflammation.

In addition to the inflammatory changes seen in allergic disease, common pathophysiologic mechanisms are noted in both CRS and asthma. In each of these diseases, as well as in allergic rhinitis, the primary effector cell is the eosinophil.[20] In both CRS and asthma, progressive inflammatory changes occur in the epithelium over time, involving elements of basement membrane thickening, goblet cell hyperplasia, cellular infiltration, and mucus hypersecretion.[21] The coexistence of asthma and CRS seems to be associated with worse pathophysiologic mucosal changes in both the sinuses and the lungs than is seen with either disease alone.[22] Although remodeling is seen in both patients with CRS and those with asthma, the degree of remodeling seems to be less in the nose than in the lung.[23] However, the generalized presence of inflammatory mediators throughout the respiratory tract shows that communication occurs between portions of the respiratory system on both a cellular and a mediator level.[11]

The interactive effects of nasal inflammation and lower airway physiology have been shown clinically in several studies. Several articles have shown that direct nasal antigen or irritant challenge can result in a significant increase in bronchial hyperreactivity.[24,25] In addition, the severity of asthma symptoms worsens directly with increasing rhinitis, supporting the role of nasal inflammation in exacerbating lower airway disease.[26] Furthermore, treatment of allergic rhinitis with topical intranasal corticosteroids is associated with decrease in asthma symptoms and improvement in objective indices of pulmonary function.[25,27,28] In addition, both medical and surgical management of CRS have been shown to decrease asthma symptoms and to decrease inflammatory mediators in the lower airway.[13,29,30]

In addition to direct effects with medical and surgical management, treatment of allergic rhinitis with subcutaneous immunotherapy has been shown to not only improve rhinitis symptoms, but to also downregulate systemic inflammatory mediators and reduce asthma symptoms.[31,32] Because concurrent disease in both the upper and lower airways is common, immunomodulatory therapy can promote system-wide beneficial effects, not only in the reduction of rhinitis symptoms but in the improvement of asthma symptoms and asthma control.

An evaluation of these various clinical studies confirms the close association of the upper and lower airway in health and disease. Shared inflammatory processes are at the core of this respiratory interdependence, and factors that increase symptoms in one portion of the airway generally result in increased disease throughout the airway. Direct influences on the nasal airway, including nasal congestion and nasal obstruction, can further exacerbate these symptoms, contributing to not only nasal disease but to worsening asthma symptoms as well.

## NASAL SURGERY AND THE UNIFIED AIRWAY
### Rhinitis and Asthma

Rhinitis is a common disorder, affecting 20% to 30% of the population. Among patients with rhinitis, as many as 40% have concurrent asthma. In contrast with the prevalence of asthma in the general population, which is about 7%, there is a much higher proportion of patients with rhinitis who have asthma. As a result, facial plastic surgeons should be alert to the potential presence of asthma in their surgical patients, many of whom may have rhinitis, and should query these patients about asthma symptoms such as cough, wheezing, and shortness of breath. Because asthma is a risk during general anesthesia, patients need to have achieved maximal asthma control at the time of their surgical treatment, especially in elective surgical cases.

### Nasal Packing

One consideration in nasal surgery, for both septoplasty and rhinoplasty, is the use of nasal packing. Packing has traditionally been used to decrease bleeding following nasal surgery, to prevent the formation of septal hematoma, and to protect the positioning of the septum in the early postoperative period. Not all nasal surgeons use nasal packing, and some use it selectively based on patient factors at the time of surgery. In addition, some nasal packing materials are not totally occlusive, being designed with small ventilation tubes in the center of the packs.

In one recent study, the use of both ventilated and totally occlusive nasal packs was studied in patients who underwent both septoplasty and septorhinoplasty.[33] In this study, the investigators randomly assigned surgical patients to receive postoperative packing with either occlusive or ventilated packs, and assessed their cardiac function and arterial blood gases after surgery. Results showed that patients receiving totally occlusive packs had significant decreases in $HCO_3$ and $pCO_2$ concentrations in the arterial blood, without effects on pH or oxygenation, which the investigators attributed to increased ventilatory rate. In addition, patients in both groups showed changes in heart rate variability as measured by Holter monitor. The investigators thought that nasal packing caused vagally stimulated cardiac changes, and warned that packing should be used with caution in elderly patients, especially individuals with underlying cardiopulmonary disease. In addition, they suggested that nasal packs with airways are preferable in patients susceptible to hypoxia. In other studies comparing nasal packs with and without airways, $O_2$ saturation was noted to be lower in patients receiving totally occlusive packs than in patients treated with ventilated nasal packs.[34,35] The investigators in the former study noted that, in elderly patients and those with chronic obstructive pulmonary disease (COPD), the presence of an airway tube in the nasal packing seemed to reduce the risk of hypoxia. Additional studies have cautioned surgeons about the potential risks of nasal packing. In several studies, nasal packing has been shown to decrease arterial $pO_2$ and increase arterial $pCO_2$, suggesting decreased ventilation secondary to the packs.[36–38]

Although none of the aforementioned studies specifically evaluated patients with asthma, it seems that occlusive nasal packs might be of greater risk in the asthmatic patient than in the general population, and care should be taken in their use among this population. Among the elderly, as well as those with obstructive pulmonary disease, there seems to be increased risk with totally occluding nasal packs. It is therefore wise for facial plastic surgeons to take into consideration these factors when deciding whether or not to place nasal packs in a patient, as well as whether the use of ventilated nasal packing may decrease the risk of hypoxia and cardiac arrhythmia in susceptible individuals.

## Air Inspiration

As noted previously, nasal conditioning of inspired air is critical in the delivery of appropriately warmed and humidified air to the lower airway. The inspiration of cold, dry air is associated with increased pulmonary resistance and bronchial hyperreactivity. Among patients with asthma, therefore, facilitation of effective nasal breathing is important in decreasing asthma symptoms and improving pulmonary function. Corrective septal surgery is associated with improvement in conditioning of inspired air,[39] which permits improved airflow quality to the lower airways, and potentially improves pulmonary function.

Although surgery on the nose can improve nasal function and conditioning of inspired air, mention must be made of the risk of aggressive turbinate resection and its effects on decreasing humidification and temperature control in the nasal cavity. Aggressive turbinate reduction can be associated with adverse physiologic effects on the nose.[40] Chronic crusting, atrophic rhinitis, and perception of inadequate airflow are associated with aggressive turbinate surgery and, as a result, more conservative procedures are currently used. The worst representation of this aggressive surgery is seen in the so-called empty-nose syndrome, in which both the inferior and middle turbinates are often totally removed, resulting in a widely patent, but dysfunctional, nasal airway. Although inferior turbinectomy has been recommended as a component of rhinoplasty surgery, its current use cannot be supported because of the significant number of patients who experience symptoms of excessive dryness and atrophic rhinitis. Concerning its risk on the unified airway; these changes in normal physiologic conditioning of inspired air are potentially associated with increased risk of lower airway symptoms and pulmonary dysfunction.

## IMPLICATIONS OF THE UNIFIED AIRWAY MODEL

The unified airway model documents the strong anatomic and physiologic associations between the upper and lower respiratory tracts, and highlights the interdependence of the entire respiratory system in health and disease. Given the implications of the unified airway model, there are 2 areas that deserve specific consideration by the facial plastic surgeon in the planning of septoplasty and rhinoplasty:

1. Preoperative evaluation of the patient undergoing nasal surgery

## 2. Management of the nose in the perioperative and postoperative periods

Because many patients seeking treatment from otolaryngologists and facial plastic surgeons have complaints of nasal airway obstruction and congestion, it is important for surgeons to appreciate the close association between both allergic and nonallergic rhinitis and asthma. Because prevalence rates for asthma in this population approach 40%, many patients seeking surgical treatment of rhinitis symptoms may have underlying asthma, which may or may not be diagnosed at the time of presentation. It is important to realize that cough, especially nighttime cough, among patients with allergic rhinitis may reflect underlying asthmatic bronchospasm, even among patients without wheezing or dyspnea. In addition, exercise intolerance or wheezing with exercise may also reflect intermittent asthma among otherwise healthy young adults. Facial plastic surgeons should inquire about cough-induced and exercise-induced dyspnea and wheezing among their preoperative patients, especially among patients with significant symptoms of rhinitis. If the patient's history suggests the presence of asthma, further evaluation with pulmonary function testing would be useful, as well as consideration of referral to a pulmonary specialist, otolaryngic allergist, or allergist/immunologist who might assist with diagnosis and management. Because asthma can present an increased anesthetic risk, communication with the anesthesiologist concerning the presence of asthma is essential in mitigating any unnecessary risk and in allowing perioperative management with bronchodilators and/or corticosteroids to maximize intraoperative pulmonary function.

At the completion of nasal surgery, the facial plastic surgeon makes a decision about the potential use of nasal packing during the postoperative period. Placement of nasal packs is based on many factors, as discussed previously. There is an extensive literature that shows the adverse effects of nasal packing on oxygenation, ventilation, and cardiac rate and rhythm. Although nasal packs may be tolerated without incident in healthy adults, they can potentially present an issue in elderly patients, patients with underlying obstructive pulmonary disease, and patients with a history of cardiac disease and arrhythmia. In these susceptible individuals, packing should be used judiciously, if at all, and, among patients thought to be at significant increased risk, consideration should be given to overnight monitoring in an inpatient setting for at least the first night following surgery if nasal packing is required.

Packing materials that incorporate an airway tube may lessen some of these risks slightly, but it seems that all nasal packs are associated with increased risk of cardiopulmonary events among susceptible patients. These factors should be considered as part of the preoperative evaluation of patients undergoing nasal surgery, and appropriate planning and consent should be used.

## SUMMARY

There is growing recognition that the upper and lower respiratory tracts function as an interdependent physiologic mechanism, and that stimuli that trigger pathophysiologic changes in one portion of the airway can provoke similar changes throughout the airway. The unified airway model acknowledges these shared airway features, suggesting the importance of comprehensive evaluation of patients with any respiratory symptoms. An appreciation of these relationships is important for the facial plastic surgeon performing elective septoplasty and rhinoplasty, and consideration and management of potential cardiopulmonary risks among susceptible individuals is vital in the appropriate perioperative management of these patients.

## REFERENCES

1. Krouse JH. The unified airway – conceptual framework. Otolaryngol Clin N Am 2008;41:257–66.
2. Braunstahl GJ, Hellings PW. Nasobronchial interaction mechanisms in allergic airway disease. Curr Opin Otolaryngol Head Neck Surg 2006;14:176–82.
3. Krouse JH, Veling MC, Ryan MW, et al. Executive summary: asthma and the unified airway. Otolaryngol Head Neck Surg 2007;136:699–706.
4. Passalacqua G, Ciprandi G, Canonica GW. United airway disease: therapeutic aspects. Thorax 2000; 55:S26–7.
5. Bousquet J, van Cauwenberge P, Khaltaev N, et al. Allergic Rhinitis and its Impact on Asthma (ARIA): executive summary of the workshop report. Allergy 2002;57:841–55.
6. Brozek JL, Bousquet J, Baena-Cagnani CE, et al. Allergic Rhinitis and its Impact on Asthma (ARIA) guidelines: 2010 revision. J Allergy Clin Immunol 2010;126:466–76.
7. Guerra S, Sherrill DL, Martinez FD, et al. Rhinitis as an independent risk factor for adult-onset asthma. J Allergy Clin Immunol 2002;109:419–25.
8. Settipane GA, Greisner WA 3rd, Settipane RJ. Natural history of asthma: a 23-year follow-up of college students. Ann Allergy Asthma Immunol 2000;84:499–503.

9. Corren J. Allergic rhinitis and asthma: how important is the link? J Allergy Clin Immunol 1997;99:S781–6.

10. European Community Respiratory Health Survey II Steering Committee. The European Community Respiratory Health Survey II. Eur Respir J 2002;20: 1071–9.

11. Jani A, Hamilos D. Current thinking on the relationship between rhinosinusitis and asthma. J Asthma 2005;42:1–7.

12. Senior B, Kennedy D, Tanabodee J. Long-term impact of functional endoscopic sinus surgery on asthma. Otolaryngol Head Neck Surg 1999;121: 66–8.

13. Batra P, Kern R, Tripathi A, et al. Outcome analysis of endoscopic sinus surgery in patients with nasal polyps and asthma. Laryngoscope 2003;113: 1703–6.

14. Shturman-Ellstein R, Zeballos RJ, Buckley JM, et al. The beneficial effect of nasal breathing on exercise-induced bronchoconstriction. Am Rev Respir Dis 1978;118:65–73.

15. Fisher LH, Davies MJ, Craig TJ. Nasal obstruction, the airway, and the athlete. Clin Rev Allergy Immunol 2005;29:151–8.

16. Helenius I, Haahtala T. Allergy and asthma in elite summer sport athletes. J Allergy Clin Immunol 2000;106:444–52.

17. Ogura JH, Harvey JE. Nasopulmonary mechanics – experimental evidence of the influence of the upper airway upon the lower. Acta Otolaryngol 1971;71: 123–32.

18. Ogura JH, Togawa K, Dammkoehler R. Nasal obstruction and the mechanics of breathing: physiologic relationships and effects of nasal surgery. Arch Otolaryngol 1966;83:135–50.

19. Cassi NJ, Biller HF, Ogura JH. Changes in arterial oxygen tension and pulmonary mechanisms with use of posterior packing in epistaxis. Laryngoscope 1971;81:1261–6.

20. Ponikau J, Sherris D, Kephart G, et al. Features of airway remodeling and eosinophilic inflammation in chronic rhinosinusitis: is the histopathology similar to asthma? J Allergy Clin Immunol 2003;112:877–82.

21. Bachert C, Vignola M, Gevaert P, et al. Allergic rhinitis, rhinosinusitis, and asthma: one airway disease. Immunol Allergy Clin N Am 2004;24:19–43.

22. Dhong H, Hyo K, Cho D. Histopathological characteristics of chronic sinusitis with bronchial asthma. Acta Otolaryngol 2005;125:169–76.

23. Braunstahl GJ, Fokkens WJ, Overbeek SE, et al. Mucosal and systemic inflammatory changes in allergic rhinitis and asthma: a comparison between upper and lower airways. Clin Exp Allergy 2003;33: 579–87.

24. Littell NT, Carlisle CC, Millman RP, et al. Changes in airway resistance following nasal provocation. Am Rev Respir Dis 1990;141:580–3.

25. Corren J, Adinoff AD, Irvin CG. Changes in bronchial responsiveness following nasal provocation with allergen. J Allergy Clin Immunol 1992; 89:611–8.

26. Corren J. The impact of allergic rhinitis on bronchial asthma. J Allergy Clin Immunol 1998;101:S352–6.

27. Welsh PW, Stricker WE, Chu CP, et al. Efficacy of beclomethasone nasal solution, flunisolide, and cromolyn in relieving symptoms of ragweed allergy. Mayo Clin Proc 1987;62:125–34.

28. Watson WT, Becker AB, Simons FE. Treatment of allergic rhinitis with intranasal corticosteroids in patients with mild asthma: effect on lower airway responsiveness. J Allergy Clin Immunol 1993;91: 97–101.

29. Ikeda K, Tanno N, Tamura G, et al. Endoscopic sinus surgery improves pulmonary function in patients with asthma associated with chronic sinusitis. Ann Otol Rhinol Laryngol 1999;108:355–9.

30. Ragab S, Scadding GK, Lund VJ, et al. Treatment of chronic rhinosinusitis and its effect on asthma. Eur Respir J 2006;28:68–74.

31. Walker SM, Pajno GB, Lima MT, et al. Grass pollen immunotherapy for seasonal rhinitis and asthma: a randomized, controlled trial. J Allergy Clin Immunol 2001;107:87–93.

32. Passalacqua G, Durham SR. Allergic rhinitis and its impact on asthma update: allergen immunotherapy. J Allergy Clin Immunol 2007;119:881–91.

33. Zeyyan E, Bajin MD, Aytemir K, et al. The effects on cardiac functions and arterial blood gases of totally occluding nasal packs and nasal packs with airway. Laryngoscope 2010;120: 2325–30.

34. Erpek G, Yorulmaz A. Nasal packing and nocturnal oxygen saturations. KBB ve Bas Boyun Cerrahisi Dergisi 1997;5:209–11.

35. Yigit O, Cinar U, Uslu B, et al. Effects of nasal packs with and without airway on nocturnal blood gases. KBB Ihtis Derg 2002;9:347–50.

36. Cook TA, Komorn RM. Statistical analysis of the alterations of blood gases produced by nasal packing. Laryngoscope 1973;83:1802–9.

37. Jacobs JR, Levine LA, Davis H. Posterior packs and the nasopulmonary reflex. Laryngoscope 1981;91: 279–84.

38. Solcum CW, Maisel RH, Cantrell RW. Arterial blood gases determination in patients with anterior packing. Laryngoscope 1976;86:869–73.

39. Wiesmiller K, Keck T, Rettinger G, et al. Nasal air conditioning in patients before and after septoplasty with bilateral turbinoplasty. Laryngoscope 2006;116: 890–4.

40. Moore GF, Freeman TJ, Ogren FP, et al. Extended follow-up of total inferior turbinate resection for relief of chronic nasal obstruction. Laryngoscope 1985; 95:1095–9.

# Pharmacotherapy of Rhinitis and Rhinosinusitis

Mohamad Chaaban, MD*, Jacquelynne P. Corey, MD

## KEYWORDS

- Rhinitis • Rhinosinusitis • Pharmacotherapy • Allergy
- Allergic conjunctivitis

---

### Key Points

- Intranasal corticosteroids (INCS) are an effective first-line treatment of allergic rhinitis.
- INCS are more effective than oral antihistamines or leukotriene receptor antagonists for the treatment of allergic rhinitis.
- Intranasal antihistamines are effective for nasal congestion and some types of nonallergic rhinitis.
- Most oral antihistamines control all the nasal symptoms of rhinitis except nasal congestion.
- Topical antihistamines, mast cell stabilizers, or combinations are useful for allergic rhinoconjunctivitis (ARC).
- Ocular itching is the pathognomonic sign of ARC.
- The most common bacteria isolated from the maxillary sinuses of patients with acute bacterial rhinosinusitis include *Streptococcus pneumoniae*, *Haemophilus influenzae*, and *Moraxella catarrhalis*.
- Most guidelines recommend amoxicillin as first-line therapy for the treatment of acute rhinosinusitis because of its safety, effectiveness, low cost, and narrow microbiological spectrum.
- A 2009 Cochrane review suggested the use of INCS as a monotherapy or as an adjunct to antibiotics for patients with acute rhinosinusitis.
- Cosmetic surgery in patients with inflammation due to ARC, acute rhinosinusitis, or chronic rhinosinusitis may be performed if treatment, avoidance, or timing is used to reduce inflammation.

---

Symptomatic allergic rhinoconjunctivitis (ARC) affects around 20% of adults in the United States. A nationwide survey in 2006 showed that 54.6% of people in the United States tested positive for at least 1 allergen.[1] Allergic disorders can affect all portions of the respiratory tree, including the nose, and commonly affect the eyes as well. Concerns for the cosmetic surgeon relative to allergic disorders include diagnosis, treatment, and assessment of the disease and whether or not therapy may affect the timing or outcome of cosmetic procedures. In this article, the pharmacotherapy of allergic and nonallergic rhinoconjunctivitis and rhinosinusitis is discussed. Although rhinitis and conjunctivitis may both occur without IgE mediated allergy, it is the most common mechanism. Rhinosinusitis, both acute and chronic, involves inflammation, which may be reduced with antiinflammatory therapies.

## PATHOPHYSIOLOGY OF ARC

Allergen sensitization in the nose starts with the interaction of the antigen-presenting cell with the

---

Department of Surgery, Section of Otolaryngology–Head and Neck Surgery, University of Chicago Medical Center, 5841 South Maryland Avenue, Chicago, IL 60637, USA
* Corresponding author.
*E-mail address:* mchaaban@gmail.com

Facial Plast Surg Clin N Am 20 (2012) 61–71
doi:10.1016/j.fsc.2011.10.007
1064-7406/12/$ – see front matter © 2012 Elsevier Inc. All rights reserved.

T helper cell. On deposition of the allergen in a susceptible host, the interaction results in IgE production (**Fig. 1**).[2] This IgE response is the pathophysiologic basis of allergic rhinitis, and it includes both early and late phases. The most important cell mediating the early response is the mast cell. Cross-linkage of membrane-bound IgE triggers mast cell degranulation, releasing histamine and a cascade of allergic and inflammatory mediators. During the early phase, there may be symptoms of itchiness, rhinorrhea, and sneezing. In the late phase, B cells (T cells and basophils) are recruited. The presence of these cells results in an increase in production of allergen-specific IgE and increased hyperresponsiveness to the allergen.

## DIAGNOSIS OF RHINITIS
### History

Documenting the patient's history is the most important first step. The patient should be encouraged to describe specific symptoms, such as sneezing, itchy eyes, and nasal blockage. Common allergic symptoms include nasal blockage/congestion; rhinorrhea (anterior and posterior); paranasal pain or headache; sneezing; pruritus; itchy, watery, or red eyes; anosmia; dysosmia; chronic pharyngitis; and hoarseness. Symptoms may occur perennially from dust mites, molds, cockroaches, cats, or dogs and/or seasonally from trees, grasses, weeds, and seasonal molds.

Patients with allergy generally have many concurrent symptoms. It is important to ask the patient to focus on what is most bothersome and choose the 3 to 4 most prominent symptoms, such as nasal congestion, itchy eyes, sneezing, and red eyes.

Physicians should document the factors that worsen symptoms, such as windy days for pollen or visits to a home with pets; medications being used, both prescription and over-the-counter (OTC); and the patient's response or lack of response to the treatments. It should be noted that many allergy medications are available OTC at present, and most patients have tried at least OTC treatment or received a prescription from their primary care physician. A family history of documented allergy can be an important clue that current symptoms may be caused by allergy. It is also important to ask about other related health issues, including atopic disorders such as eczema, food allergy and uriticaria.

### Physical Examination

Initial examination can show classic signs of allergy, such as "boggy" bluish nasal mucosa, red inflamed nasal mucosa, or excessive clear watery mucus. In the eyes, dark skin of the lower eyelids (allergic shiners), periorbital and/or conjunctival erythema, and edema may be present.

Seasonal and perennial allergic conjunctivitis represent most cases of ocular allergy, whereas the more severe conditions of atopic keratoconjunctivitis (AKC) and vernal keratoconjunctivitis (VKC) affect a smaller group of patients. **Fig. 2** shows photographs of eyes from individuals with the various forms of allergic conjunctivitis.[3] Allergic conjunctivitis is typically elicited by ocular exposure to allergen. Despite differences in

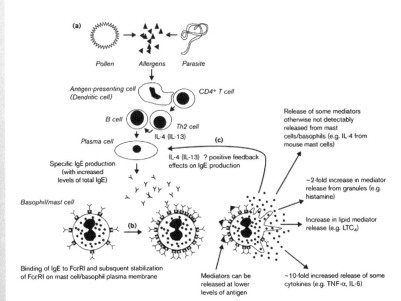

Fig. 1. (a) Various factors can trigger immune responses, whereby specific IgE is produced by plasma cells. (b) Binding of IgE upregulates its receptors and results in response at lower levels of antigen (eg, allergens) and in increased release of mediators and cytokines. (c) There may also be a positive feedback via IL-4 and IL-13 that increases IgE production. (*Adapted from* Wedemeyer J, Tsai M, Galli SJ. Roles of mast cells and basophils in innate and acquired immunity. Curr Opin Immunol 2000; 12(6):627; with permission.)

Seasonal Allergic Conjunctivitis

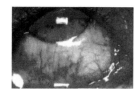

Vernal Keratoconjunctivitis

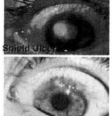
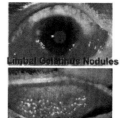

Atopic Keratoconjunctivitis

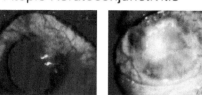

Giant Papillary Conjunctivitis

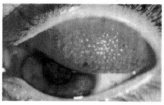

**Fig. 2.** Types of allergic conjunctivitis. (*Adapted from* Ono SJ, Abelson MB. Allergic conjunctivitis: update on pathophysiology and prospects for future treatment. J Allergy Clin Immunol 2005;115(1):119; with permission.)

disease classification and incidence, the allergic response in conjunctivitis is similar to the pathophysiology of allergic rhinitis. The pathognomonic symptom of ocular allergy is itching. Most patients with allergic rhinitis also have eye symptoms.[4,5]

### Testing

Various testing methods are used for allergic disorders, including skin prick, intradermal testing, serial dilution titration, and in vitro allergy tests. Practitioners who do not practice immunotherapy in their office may wish to confirm diagnoses through in vitro testing for allergen-specific IgE of common allergens after a trial of appropriate pharmacotherapy.

### TREATMENT OPTIONS FOR RHINITIS AND RHINOSINUSITIS

There are multiple types of treatments for ARC, including avoidance of known initiating triggers, pharmacotherapy, and immunotherapy. However, the only treatment that has been shown to alter the natural history of this disease is immunotherapy. In this article, the treatment is discussed in 3 broad categories: avoidance, pharmacotherapy, and immunotherapy. Allergic conjunctivitis is treated similarly, although immunotherapy is rarely indicated for allergic conjunctivitis alone.

### Avoidance

Patients with ARC may benefit from avoiding inciting factors, effectively reducing symptoms. It may be difficult for patients to comply with the

recommendations because they may interfere with their daily life activities. Patients allergic to house dust mites can use allergen-impermeable encasings on the bed and pillows. Pollen exposure can be reduced by keeping windows closed, using an air conditioner, and limiting the amount of time spent outdoors.[6] Avoiding basements and reducing household humidity is important in patients who have mold allergy. Filtration systems, including high-efficiency particulate air filters, may be used to aid in decreasing the allergen load.[7] Patients who are allergic to pets should avoid having pets in the house or at least in their bedroom. The effectiveness of avoidance measures may be small because of the ubiquity of inhalant allergens.[2,8] However, reports of individual patient responses vary, and the diligent use of multiple avoidance measures simultaneously with medical therapy can be beneficial.

### PHARMACOTHERAPY OF ALLERGIC RHINITIS

Symptoms may be generally divided into 2 broad categories: runners and blockers. Runners complain of rhinorrhea; sneezing; itchy nose, eyes, and throat; and red eyes. These symptoms are related mostly to early-phase mediators, such as histamine, and respond well to oral or intranasal antihistamines and steroids. Blockers usually complain of nasal congestion and benefit from intranasal steroids, leukotriene inhibitors, and intranasal antihistamines.

There are 2 broad categories of pharmacologic treatments for patients with allergic rhinitis. The targeted forms of treatment are drugs that act on the mediators of the mast cell, whereas immuno-modulatory therapies prevent initiation and/or downregulate the immunologic response.[2]

Targeted therapies include decongestants, antihistamines, anticholinergics, leukotriene inhibitors, and mast cell stabilizers. Immunomodulators include mast cell stabilizers, leukotriene inhibitors, steroids (oral, intranasal, ophthalmic, or depot injection), and allergen-specific IgE treatment (either subcutaneous or sublingual) or anti-IgE injection (omalizumab).

## Intranasal Corticosteroids

The mainstay of treatment of allergic rhinitis is intranasal corticosteroids (INCS). Their mechanism of action is to inhibit the release of cytokines, decrease inflammatory cells, and reduce inflammation of the nasal mucosa.[9] Steroids have an onset of action of about 30 minutes, with their peak effect taking hours to days and their maximum effect usually taking 2 to 4 weeks.[10]

Initial indications for INCS included second-line or add-on treatment of ARC. New data show that INCS are more effective than oral or intranasal antihistamines for the treatment of allergic rhinitis, justifying first-line treatment.[8,10–12] **Table 1** shows a list of some of the commonly used intranasal steroids with their brand names and potential side effects, which include bitter aftertaste, burning, epistaxis, headache, nasal dryness, potential risk of systemic absorption, rhinitis medicamentosa, stinging, and throat irritation.[10,12]

**Table 1**
**INCS**

| Generic Name | Brand Name | Dosage |
| --- | --- | --- |
| Beclomethasone | Beconase | 1–2 puffs each side, bid |
| Budesonide | Rhinocort | 1–4 puffs each side, qd |
| Ciclesonide | Omnaris | 1–2 puffs each side, qd |
| Fluticasone propionate | Flonase[a] | 1–2 puffs each side, qd |
| Fluticasone furoate | Veramyst | 1–2 puffs each side, qd |
| Mometasone | Nasonex | 1–2 puffs each side, qd |
| Triamcinolone | Nasacort | 1–2 puffs each side, qd |

*Abbreviations:* bid, twice daily; qd, every day.
[a] Generic available.

The potential for cataract formation and glaucoma may be a concern for the cosmetic surgeon. Current literature indicates that there is very little evidence of an association between INCS and glaucoma or cataract formation.[13] There is no evidence in the literature to support the usage of any particular INCS because they have not been shown to be different except for their age indications in accordance with the US Food and Drug Administration (FDA).[14–16]

## Oral and Topical Antihistamines

Antihistamines can be used for the treatment of ARC. They can be used as oral or topical treatments. Oral antihistamines include first-generation and second-generation antihistamines. The first-generation antihistamines are more lipid soluble and are able to cross the blood-brain barrier more readily than those of the second generation. For this reason, first-generation antihistamines have been associated with adverse effects, including, but not limited to, sedation, fatigue, impaired mental status, poor school performance, impaired driving, and increase in automobile collisions and work-related injuries.[17–20] Common first-generation and second-generation oral antihistamines are listed in **Table 2**.[21–23] Most second-generation antihistamines have a more complex chemical structure, thus decreasing their capability to cross the blood-brain barrier. For this reason, most second-generation antihistamines have very low sedation potential and central nervous system side effects, and are therefore considered nonsedating. Oral cetirizine and oral levocetirizine, intranasal azelastine, and intranasal olopatadine have a lower sedation potential than first-generation antihistamines but are not classified as nonsedating. Most oral antihistamines control nasal and ocular symptoms with minimal effect on nasal congestion, with the exception of desloratadine.[24] Because of their rapid onset of action (between 15 and 30 minutes) and their safety for use in children older than 6 months, antihistamines are frequently used for mild symptoms requiring as-needed treatment.[2]

The advantages of topical antihistamines over oral antihistamines include utility in controlling nasal congestion. This effect may be due to delivery of a higher concentration of the drug on the target organ or a mild antiinflammatory effect.[21] Some of the topical antihistamines may have a bitter taste (10% of subjects). Topical antihistamines have a slightly higher incidence of drowsiness (10%) than the nonsedating oral antihistamines. Intranasal antihistamines include azelastine (Astelin), azelastine hydrochloride

## Table 2
### First-generation and second-generation oral antihistamines with commonly used doses for adults

| Generic Name | Brand Name | Dosage |
| --- | --- | --- |
| First generation | | |
| Dexchlorpheniramine[a] | Polaramine | 2 mg po q 4–6 h |
| Diphenhydramine[a] | Benadryl | 25 mg po q 4–6 h |
| Hydroxyzine | Atarax | 25–100 mg po q 4–8 h |
| Promethazine | Phenergan | 12.5–25 mg po q 6–24 h |
| Second generation | | |
| Cetirizine[a] | Zyrtec | 5–10 mg po qd |
| Desloratadine | Clarinex | 5 mg po qd |
| Fexofenadine[a] | Allegra | 180 mg po qd or 60 mg po bid |
| Levocetirizine | Xyzal | 5 mg po qd |
| Loratadine[a] | Claritin | 10 mg po qd |

Abbreviations: bid, twice daily; po, per oral; q, every; qd, every day.

[a] Available OTC.

Data from Refs.[21–23]

(Astepro), and olopatadine (Patanase) and are approved for the treatment of ARC. Their onset of action occurs within 15 minutes and lasts up to 12 hours. Other potential side effects include headache, nasal irritation, and epistaxis.[21,22,25]

Topical ocular treatments of allergic conjunctivitis include antihistamines, mast cell stabilizers, and combination antihistamine/mast cell stabilizers. Topical ophthalmic steroids are also available, but their use is limited for simple perennial allergic rhinitis; an ophthalmologist's consultation may be needed for other types of ARCs, such as AKC or VKC. An example of an ocular antihistamine is emedastine dirfurmarate (Emadine). Common ocular antihistamine/mast cell–stabilizing combinations used include olopatadine hydrochloride (Patanol), olopatadine hydrochloride (Pataday), epinastine hydrochloride (Elestat), azelastine hydrochloride (Optivar), and ketotifen fumarate (Zaditor), an OTC medication. There are ocular mast cell stabilizers that include first-generation and second-generation drugs; because these are more potent, second-generation drugs can be dosed less frequently. The first-generation ocular mast cell stabilizers include lodoxamide (Alomide) and cromolyn sodium (Crolom). Second-generation drugs include nedocromil sodium (Alocril) or pemirolast potassium (Alamast).[26]

## Decongestants

Oral and topical decongestants may be used for patients with allergic rhinitis. These decongestants act by causing vasoconstriction in the nasal mucosa, subsequently resulting in decreased swelling. Pseudoephedrine used for 2 weeks showed relief of symptoms. The most commonly available decongestants are topical phenylephrine (Neo-Synephrine), topical oxymetazoline (Afrin), and oral pseudoephedrine (Sudafed). The use of intranasal decongestants should be limited to no more than 3 to 5 days because of the risk of developing rhinitis medicamentosa or rebound congestion.[23] Patients with underlying cardiovascular conditions, hypertension, glaucoma, or hyperthyroidism should be very careful in using these medications[11,25] because they may cause headache, elevated blood pressure, tremor, urinary retention, dizziness, tachycardia, or insomnia. Many oral antihistamines have been combined with an oral decongestant to relieve nasal congestion.[8,11,25]

## Intranasal Cromolyn

Intranasal cromolyn inhibits degranulation of mast cells. It is generally safe and available OTC. This drug is generally given 3 to 4 times daily, with decreased effectiveness at relieving symptoms compared with either intranasal steroids or antihistamines.[27,28]

## Intranasal Anticholinergics

Intranasal anticholinergics are useful for excessive rhinorrhea. The drug that is most commonly used is ipratropium bromide (Atrovent, intranasal). It needs to be administered 2 or 3 times daily. The drug does not cross the blood-brain barrier and is not systemically absorbed. The potential adverse side effects include, but are not limited to, dryness of the nasal mucosa, epistaxis, and headache.[27]

## Leukotriene Receptor Antagonists

Because leukotrienes C4, D4, and E4 are part of the early and rapid de novo generation of mediators in the early phase of allergic rhinitis, developing drugs that affect their activity is useful.

These mediators are believed to produce nasal congestion symptoms. Although better than placebo, leukotriene receptor antagonists are suggested as either second-line or third-line therapy. Montelukast (Singulair), a leukotriene $LTD_4$ receptor antagonist, is approved for the treatment of allergic rhinitis and asthma.[29–31]

### Combination Therapy

Monotherapy with intranasal steroids has been shown to be generally as effective for nasal symptoms as combinations of either oral antihistamine or leukotriene receptor antagonists with intranasal steroids. Fluticasone together with azelastine has been shown to be superior to treatment with intranasal steroids alone for patients with moderate to severe allergic rhinitis.[12,32–34] To aid in additional relief or more rapid relief of eye symptoms, it may be reasonable for patients with severe symptoms to have combination therapy. The results of a systematic review, together with data on safety and cost-effectiveness, support the use of INCS over oral antihistamines as first-line treatment of allergic rhinitis.[10]

## ALLERGEN IMMUNOTHERAPY

Subcutaneous allergen immunotherapy can be highly effective in controlling symptoms of allergic rhinitis and favorably modifies the long-term course of the disease.[35] Patients with allergic rhinitis should be considered candidates for immunotherapy on the basis of the severity of their symptoms, failure or unacceptability of other treatment modalities, the presence of comorbid conditions, and possibly as a means of preventing worsening of the condition or the development of comorbid conditions (eg, asthma and sinusitis).[36,37] Approximately 80% or more of patients experience symptomatic improvement after 1 to 2 years of subcutaneous immunotherapy; current guidelines recommend that treatment be continued for 4 to 5 years.[38] Allergen immunotherapy for ARC can reduce the development of asthma in children and possibly in adults.[38–40] Sublingual immunotherapy is a more recently developed form of immunotherapy and is popular in Europe.[41]

## PHARMACOTHERAPY OF NONALLERGIC RHINITIS
### FDA-Approved Treatments

Vasomotor rhinitis is a term that is sometimes used synonymously with the term nonallergic rhinitis without eosinophilia. It is often used to describe the condition in which patients exhibit hyperreactivity to nonallergic triggers that are not mediated by allergen-specific IgE.[28,39] Examples of conditions causing this hyperreactivity include, but are not limited to, temperature changes, changes in relative humidity, odors, tobacco smoke, alcohol, sexual arousal, and emotional factors.[42] There are several drugs used to treat nonallergic rhinitis. Azelastine is an intranasal antihistamine approved for the treatment of nonallergic rhinitis. Budesonide is approved for long-term therapy in nonallergic rhinitis.[43] Treatment using intranasal cromoglycate showed improvement in symptoms of nonallergic rhinitis.[44]

### Non-FDA–Approved Treatments

Ipratropium bromide is useful for nonallergic rhinorrhea, such as skier's nose or food-induced rhinitis from spicy foods.[45,46] Some guidelines for approval of septoplasty surgery suggest that a one-month trial of INCS be attempted before the procedure; there is no scientific evidence to suggest such a trial is beneficial.[46]

## PHARMACOTHERAPY OF ACUTE SINUSITIS

Acute sinusitis is most commonly preceded by viral infections that are associated with the common cold. The pathophysiology of acute sinusitis usually consists of mucosal edema that leads to sinus ostial obstruction and impairment of ciliary function. This causes stagnation of the mucus and subsequent lowered oxygen tension, making the sinuses an excellent culture medium for viruses and bacteria.

Treatment of bacterial sinusitis can best be exemplified by the Cochrane review.[47] This review included 2 categories of trials with either antibiotics versus placebo or antibiotic versus antibiotic. The antibiotics studied included penicillin V, amoxicillin, amoxicillin/clavulanate, and azithromycin (Zithromax). When evaluating treatment with these antibiotics versus placebo for 3 to 5 days, the outcomes of cure or improvement were inconsistent. Amoxicillin/clavulanate (Augmentin) has a statistically significant lower failure rate than cephalosporins. Side effects of antibiotics are common, ranging from 8% to 59% with penicillin and 23% to 56% with amoxicillin. The most commonly reported side effects include diarrhea, abdominal pain, vomiting, and skin rash.

Antibiotics, when compared with placebo, provide a higher rate of cure and faster improvement in symptoms from acute sinusitis, but the benefit is of only modest clinical significance. For this reason, universal prescribing of antibiotics for patients with acute sinusitis could not be endorsed by the review. Available evidence does not support the broad clinical practice of prescribing antibiotics for acute sinusitis because the benefit of antibiotics is small and must be balanced with the risk of adverse effects. Watchful waiting can be considered for adults with uncomplicated acute sinusitis. Patients who are immunocompromised, have severe symptoms, or have no improvement within 7 days may benefit from antibiotics.[48]

The most common bacteria isolated from the maxillary sinuses of patients with acute bacterial rhinosinusitis (ABRS) include *Streptococcus pneumoniae*, *Haemophilus influenzae*, and *Moraxella catarrhalis*. A list of medications used for the treatment of acute sinusitis is shown on **Fig. 3**.[48] Most guidelines recommend amoxicillin as first-line therapy because of its safety, effectiveness, low cost, and narrow microbiological spectrum. Patients who are allergic to penicillin might benefit from trimethoprim/sulfamethoxazole (Bactrim, Septra) or a macrolide. When symptoms do not improve with amoxicillin therapy, then an alternative antibiotic with a broader spectrum is required. These include high-dose amoxicillin/clavulanate (Augmentin) or a respiratory fluoroquinolone.[48]

A 2009 Cochrane review suggested the use of intranasal steroids as monotherapy or as an adjunct to antibiotics for patients with acute sinusitis, although the evidence is limited.[49] Immediate evaluation and/or referral is usually required when patients have 1 of the following symptoms and/or signs: double or reduced vision, proptosis, pronounced periorbital edema, ophthalmoplegia, other focal neurologic signs, severe headache, and meningeal signs.

## PHARMACOTHERAPY OF CHRONIC RHINOSINUSITIS

Chronic sinusitis is believed to result from long-term impairment or obstruction of the sinus drainage and damage to the mucosal lining of the sinuses, which subsequently leads to a chronic low-grade bacterial infection or persistent inflammation from idiopathic causes.[50] Endoscopically directed sinus cultures taken from patients with chronic sinusitis have both aerobic and anaerobic bacteria, but it has been suggested that anaerobes play a more important role. Endoscopic cultures may be used to direct antibiotic treatment in difficult cases. Obstruction in the ostiomeatal complex is very important in the pathophysiology of sinusitis and can result from anatomic variations or mucosal inflammation.[50,51] In addition, allergy has been shown to be a contributor to the swelling and obstruction of the sinuses. Some studies suggest that sinusitis is more common in patients who are allergic than in control subjects.[52–54]

## Chronic Rhinosinusitis Without Nasal Polyposis

Intranasal steroids have been recommended for all forms of chronic rhinosinusitis (CRS), but there is insufficient evidence to demonstrate benefit for CRS without polyps.[46,55] Patients with underlying allergic rhinitis might also benefit from antihistamines.[55] If purulence is present, then antibiotics may be added, although they have not been officially approved for use in CRS. Antifungals and topical amphotericin B have been studied in patients with CRS.[56–58] Most antifungal trials have failed to show efficacy, and antifungal agents are not recommended.

## Chronic Rhinosinusitis with Nasal Polyposis

In addition to topical sprays for sinonasal polyps, a brief course of oral corticosteroids may be beneficial.[59] Mometasone (Nasonex) is indicated for polyposis as 2 puffs 2 times daily in each nostril. Studies of other drugs such as antileukotriene antagonists are limited and they are not approved for the treatment of nasal polyps. A few studies suggest that adding leukotriene inhibitors for control of sinonasal polyps may be useful (montelukast or zafirlukast) but this is inconclusive.[60] Patients who have aspirin intolerance and nasal polyposis, with aspirin-exacerbated respiratory disease, might benefit from aspirin desensitization and daily aspirin therapy, provided they have no contraindications.[61] This technique is still not widely available.

## TIMING OF COSMETIC PROCEDURES

Treatment options for allergic rhinitis and allergic conjunctivitis include avoidance measures, medications, and immunotherapy. Patients with mild symptoms, occurring for 3 months or less, can usually be treated with either avoidance or medications. Performing surgery on these patients should be avoided during their peak season; for example, avoid operating on patients allergic to ragweed from August to October. These patients should do well with surgical procedures during their off-season. Patients with moderate symptoms, or symptoms occurring for 4 to 8 months, may require 2 modalities of therapy: avoidance, medications, and/or immunotherapy. This group is the most difficult to time for cosmetic procedures because they may have very different treatment regimens, depending on whether or not they can use avoidance measures or begin immunotherapy. Patients with severe symptoms or symptoms occurring for

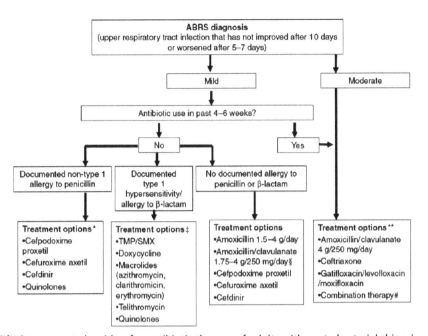

**Fig. 3.** Modified treatment algorithm for antibiotic therapy of adults with acute bacterial rhinosinusitis (ABRS) *Cephalosporins should be considered initially for patients with penicillin intolerance/non-type 1 hypersensitivity reactions (eg, rash). ‡In patients with mild disease, no recent exposure to antibiotics, and a history of beta-lactam allergies, trimethoprim/sulfamethoxazole (TMP/SMX), doxycycline, or a macrolide are recommended. §Higher daily doses of amoxicillin (4 g/day) may be advantageous in areas with a high prevalence of penicillinre-sistant Streptococcus pneumoniae or drug-resistant S pneumoniae, for patients with moderate disease, for patients who may need better Haemophilus influenzae coverage, or for patients with risk factors for infection with a resistant pathogen. There is a greater potential for treatment failure or resistant pathogens in these patient groups. **In patients with a history of beta-lactam allergies and either mild disease with recent antibiotic exposure or moderate disease, fluoroquinolones or clindamycin and rifampin are recommended. #Based on in vitro spectrum of activity, combination therapy with appropriate coverage for Gram-positive and Gram-negative pathogens may be appropriate. Examples of combination therapy regimens include high-dose amoxicillin (4 g/day) or clindamycin plus cefixime, or high-dose amoxicillin (4 g/day) or clindamycin plus rifampin. There is no clin-ical evidence at this time for the safety or efficacy of these combinations. (*Adapted from* Benninger M. Guidelines on the treatment of ABRS in adults. Int J Clin Pract 2007;61:874; with permission.)

9 months of the year or more generally require all 3 modalities to reduce the inflammatory process sufficiently and to plan cosmetic procedures safely. Medication may require 4 to 6 weeks of continuous use before inflammation and congestion are noticeably reduced. Allergen-specific immuno-therapy may take 3 to 12 months before it is effec-tive. Most patients will be taking medication and using avoidance measures concurrently. Surgical cosmetic procedures can be considered when the patient's symptoms have improved signifi-cantly and the nasal mucosal color appears normalized. Quality of life validated measures such as the Mini Rhinoconjunctivitis Quality of Life Questionnaire[62] can be used to demonstrate signif-icant improvement in symptoms.

There are limited data on performing concurrent sinus surgery and cosmetic rhinoplasty or eyelid procedures. However, septoplasty is concurrently performed with functional endoscopic sinus surgery without incident as a routine. Further study could delineate whether our common sense approach, which involves scheduling cosmetic procedures out of season or after treatment, has normalized the nasal examination to be scientifically correct.

## SUMMARY

Patients with allergic rhinitis may benefit most from intranasal steroids, which are found to be more effective than oral antihistamines, oral deconges-tants, and leukotriene receptor antagonists. Patients who have mild allergic rhinitis can use oral antihistamines on an as-needed basis. ARC may be treated with topical antihistamines, mast cell stabilizers, or combinations. Antibiotics are also helpful for patients who have nasal purulence with CRS. Cosmetic surgeons working with patients with ARC or rhinosinusitis should understand the diagnosis, treatment, and assessment of the condition to evaluate the timing and potential outcomes of relevant cosmetic procedures. The timing of cosmetic surgery may vary according to the severity of symptoms. Patients with ARC who are in season are usually advised not to undergo cosmetic procedures unless treatment has reduced inflammation to a minimum and the nasal mucosa appears to be normal. Antibiotics are indicated for patients who have acute rhinosinusitis and are immunocompromised or getting symptomatically worse.

## ACKNOWLEDGMENTS

We would like to thank Eric R. Yoo for library research and editorial assistance.

## REFERENCES

1. National Health and Nutrition Examination Survey (NHANES). Survey operations manuals, brochures, consent documents. Centers for Disease Control and Prevention (CDC). 2006. Available at: http://www.cdc.gov/nchs/nhanes/nhanes2005-2006/current_nhanes_05_06.htm. Accessed May 12, 2011.
2. Wedemeyer J, Tsai M, Galli SJ. Roles of mast cells and basophils in innate and acquired immunity. Curr Opin Immunol 2000;12(6):624–31.
3. Ono SJ, Abelson MB. Allergic conjunctivitis: update on pathophysiology and prospects for future treatment. J Allergy Clin Immunol 2005;115(1):118–22.
4. Langley KE, Patrinely JR, Anderson RL, et al. Unilateral blepharochalasis. Ophthalmic Surg 1987;18(8):594–8.
5. Lavker RM, Kligman AM. Chronic heliodermatitis: a morphologic evaluation of chronic actinic dermal damage with emphasis on the role of mast cells. J Invest Dermatol 1988;90(3):325–30.
6. van Cauwenberge P, Bachert C, Passalacqua G, et al. Consensus statement on the treatment of allergic rhinitis. Allergy 2000;55(2):116–34.
7. Ferguson BJ. Environmental control of allergens. Otolaryngol Clin N Am 2008;41:411–7.
8. Price D, Bond C, Bouchard J, et al. International Primary Care Respiratory Group (IPCRG) Guidelines: management of allergic rhinitis. Prim Care Respir J 2006;15(1):58–70.
9. Derendorf H, Meltzer EO. Molecular and clinical pharmacology of intranasal corticosteroids: clinical and therapeutic implications. Allergy 2008;63(10):1292–300.
10. Weiner JM, Abramson MJ, Puy RM. Intranasal corticosteroids versus oral H1 receptor antagonists in allergic rhinitis: systematic review of randomised controlled trials. BMJ 1998;317(7173):1624–9.
11. Scadding GK, Durham SR, Mirakian R, et al. BSACI guidelines for the management of allergic and non-allergic rhinitis. Clin Exp Allergy 2008;38(1):19–42.
12. Ratner PH, van Bavel JH, Martin BG, et al. A comparison of the efficacy of fluticasone propionate aqueous nasal spray and loratadine, alone and in combination, for the treatment of seasonal allergic rhinitis. J Fam Pract 1998;47(2):118–25.
13. Cave A, Arlett P, Lee E. Inhaled and nasal corticosteroids: factors affecting the risks of systemic adverse effects. Pharmacol Ther 1999;83(3):153–79.
14. Waddell AN, et al. Intranasal steroid sprays in the treatment of rhinitis: is one better than another? J Laryngol Otol 2003;117(11):843–5.
15. Demoly P. Safety of intranasal corticosteroids in acute rhinosinusitis. Am J Otolaryngol 2008;29(6):403–13.
16. Lumry WR. A review of the preclinical and clinical data of newer intranasal steroids used in the treatment of allergic rhinitis. J Allergy Clin Immunol 1999;104(4 Pt 1):S150–8.
17. Bender BG, Berning S, Dudden R, et al. Sedation and performance impairment of diphenhydramine and second-generation antihistamines: a meta-analysis. J Allergy Clin Immunol 2003;111(4):770–6.
18. Verster JC, Volkerts R. Antihistamines and driving ability: evidence from on-the-road driving studies during normal traffic. Ann Allergy Asthma Immunol 2004;92:294–304. Erratum in Ann Allergy Asthma Immunol 2005;94(3):409–410.
19. Corren J, Storms W, Bernstein J, et al. A systematic review of epidemiological studies investigating risk factors for work-related road traffic crashes and injuries. Inj Prev 2008;14(1):51–8.
20. Kay GG, Quig ME. Impact of sedating antihistamines on safety and productivity. Allergy Asthma Proc 2001;22(5):281–3.
21. Corren J, Storms W, Bernstein J, et al. Effectiveness of azelastine nasal spray compared with oral cetirizine in patients with seasonal allergic rhinitis. Clin Ther 2005;27(5):543–53.
22. Berger WE, White MV. Efficacy of azelastine nasal spray in patients with an unsatisfactory response to loratadine. Ann Allergy Asthma Immunol 2003;91(2):205–11.
23. Coates ML, Rembold CM, Farr BM. Does pseudoephedrine increase blood pressure in patients with controlled hypertension? J Fam Pract 1995;40(1):22–6.
24. Murdoch D, Goa KL, Keam SJ. Desloratadine: an update of its efficacy in the management of allergic disorders. Drugs 2003;63(19):2051–77.
25. Bousquet J, Van Cauwenberge P, Khaltaev N. Allergic rhinitis and its impact on asthma: ARIA workshop report. J Allergy Clin Immunol 2001;108(Suppl 5):1A–14A, S147–333.

26. Abelson MB, McLaughlin JT, Gomes PJ. Antihistamines in ocular allergy: are they all created equal? Curr Allergy Asthma Rep 2011;11(3):205–11.

27. Nelson HS, Rachelefsky GS, Bernick J. The allergy report. Milwaukee (WI): American Academy of Allergy, Asthma & Immunology; 2000.

28. Mucha SM, deTineo M, Naclerio RM, et al. Allergic rhinitis and its impact on asthma (ARIA) 2008 update (in collaboration with the World Health Organization, GA(2)LEN and AllerGen). Allergy 2008; 63(Suppl 86):8–160.

29. Grainger J, Drake-Lee A. Montelukast in allergic rhinitis: a systematic review and meta-analysis. Clin Otolaryngol 2006;31(5):360–7.

30. Wilson AM, O'Byrne PM, Parameswaran K. Leukotriene receptor antagonists for allergic rhinitis: a systematic review and meta-analysis. Am J Med 2004;116(5):338–44.

31. Juniper EF, Kline PA, Hargreave FE, et al. Comparison of montelukast and pseudoephedrine in the treatment of allergic rhinitis. Arch Otolaryngol Head Neck Surg 2006;132(2):164–72.

32. Juniper EF, et al. Comparison of beclomethasone dipropionate aqueous nasal spray, astemizole, and the combination in the prophylactic treatment of ragweed pollen-induced rhinoconjunctivitis. J Allergy Clin Immunol 1989;83(3):627–33.

33. Barnes ML, Ward JH, Fardon TC, et al. Effects of levocetirizine as add-on therapy to fluticasone in seasonal allergic rhinitis. Clin Exp Allergy 2006; 36(5):676–84.

34. Di Lorenzo G, Pacor ML, Mansueto P, et al. Randomized placebo-controlled trial comparing fluticasone aqueous nasal spray in mono-therapy, fluticasone plus cetirizine, fluticasone plus montelukast and cetirizine plus montelukast for seasonal allergic rhinitis. Clin Exp Allergy 2004;34(2):259–67.

35. Soyer OU, Akdis M, Akdis CA. Mechanisms of subcutaneous allergen immunotherapy. Immunol Allergy Clin N Am 2011;31(2):175–90.

36. Ent DV, Dykewicz MS, Bernstein DI, et al. The Joint Force on Practice Parameters, representing the AAAAI, ACAAI, JCAAI. The diagnosis and management of rhinitis: an updated practice parameter. J Allergy Clin Immunol 2008;122(Suppl): S1–84.

37. Joint Task Force on Practice Parameters; American Academy of Allergy, Asthma and Immunology; American College of Allergy, Asthma and Immunology; Joint Council of Allergy, Asthma and Immunology. Allergen immunotherapy: a practice parameter second update. J Allergy Clin Immunol 2007; 120(Suppl 3):S25–85.

38. Tam JC, Grant NL, Freire-Moran L, et al. Allergen immunotherapy: a practice parameter second update. J Allergy Clin Immunol 2007;120(Suppl 3): S25–85.

39. Wallace DV, Dykewicz MS, Bernstein DI, et al. The diagnosis and management of rhinitis: an updated practice parameter. J Allergy Clin Immunol 2008; 122(Suppl 2):S1–84.

40. Niggemann B, Jacobsen L, Dreborg S, et al. Five-year follow-up on the PAT study: specific immunotherapy and long-term prevention of asthma in children. Allergy 2006;61(7):855–9.

41. Durham SR, et al. Sublingual immunotherapy with once-daily grass allergen tablets: a randomized controlled trial in seasonal allergic rhinoconjunctivitis. J Allergy Clin Immunol 2006;117(4):802–9.

42. Dykewicz MS, Hamilos DL. Rhinitis and sinusitis. J Allergy Clin Immunol 2010;125(2 Suppl 2): S103–15.

43. Synnerstad B, Lindqvist N. A clinical comparison of intranasal budesonide with beclomethasone dipropionate for perennial non-allergic rhinitis: a 12 month study. Br J Clin Pract 1996;50(7):363–6.

44. Greiner AN, Meltzer EO. Pharmacologic rationale for treating allergic and nonallergic rhinitis. J Allergy Clin Immunol 2006;118(5):985–98.

45. Pfister SM. Ipratropium bromide (Atrovent) nasal spray. A new treatment for rhinorrhea. Nurse Pract 1996;21(7):104, 107–8.

46. Kalish LH, Arendts G, Sacks R, et al. Topical steroids in chronic rhinosinusitis without polyps: a systematic review and meta-analysis. Otolaryngol Head Neck Surg 2009;141(6):674–83.

47. Falagas ME, Giannopoulou KP, Vardakas KZ, et al. Comparison of antibiotics with placebo for treatment of acute sinusitis: a meta-analysis of randomised controlled trials. Lancet Infect Dis 2008;8(9):543–52.

48. Benninger M. Guidelines on the treatment of ABRS in adults. Int J Clin Pract 2007;61(5):873–6.

49. Zalmanovici A, Yaphe J. Steroids for acute sinusitis. Cochrane Database Syst Rev 2007;2:CD005149.

50. Frederick J, Braude AI. Anaerobic infection of the paranasal sinuses. N Engl J Med 1974;290(3):135–7.

51. Bolger WE, Butzin CA, Parsons DS. Paranasal sinus bony anatomic variations and mucosal abnormalities: CT analysis for endoscopic sinus surgery. Laryngoscope 1991;101(1 Pt 1):56–64.

52. van Dishoeck H. Allergy and infection of the paranasal sinuses. Fortschr Hals Nasen Ohrenheilkd 1961;10:1–29.

53. Pelikan Z, Pelikan-Filipek M. Role of nasal allergy in chronic maxillary sinusitis—diagnostic value of nasal challenge with allergen. J Allergy Clin Immunol 1990;86(4 Pt 1):484–91.

54. Fokkens W, Lund V, Bachert C, et al. EAACI position paper on rhinosinusitis and nasal polyps executive summary. Allergy 2005;60(5):583–601.

55. Kennedy DW, Kuhn FA, Hamilos DL, et al. Treatment of chronic rhinosinusitis with high-dose oral terbinafine: a double blind, placebo-controlled study. Laryngoscope 2005;115(10):1793–9.

56. Ponikau JU, Sherris DA, Weaver A, et al. Treatment of chronic rhinosinusitis with intranasal amphotericin B: a randomized, placebo-controlled, double-blind pilot trial. J Allergy Clin Immunol 2005;115(1):125–31.
57. Ebbens FA, Scadding GK, Badia L, et al. Amphotericin B nasal lavages: not a solution for patients with chronic rhinosinusitis. J Allergy Clin Immunol 2006; 118(5):1149–56.
58. Small CB, Hernandez J, Reyes A, et al. Efficacy and safety of mometasone furoate nasal spray in nasal polyposis. J Allergy Clin Immunol 2005;116(6): 1275–81.
59. Benítez P, Alobid I, de Haro J, et al. A short course of oral prednisone followed by intranasal budesonide is an effective treatment of severe nasal polyps. Laryngoscope 2006;116(5):770–5.
60. Modrzyński M, Zawisza E, Rapiejko P. Zafirlukast in treatment of nasal polyps in patients with aspirin intolerant bronchial asthma–preliminary report. Pol Merkur Lekarski 2002;12(69):224–7 [in Polish].
61. Williams AN, Woessner KM. The clinical effectiveness of aspirin desensitization in chronic rhinosinusitis. Curr Allergy Asthma Rep 2008;8(3):245–52.
62. Juniper EF, Thompson AK, Ferrie PJ, et al. Development and validation of the mini rhinoconjunctivitis quality of life questionnaire. Clin Exp Allergy 2000; 30(1):132–40.

# The Role of Alternative Medicine in Rhinology

Corrie E. Roehm, MD[a], Belachew Tessema, MD[a,b],
Seth M. Brown, MD, MBA[a,b],*

## KEYWORDS

- Alternative medicine • Complementary medicine
- Rhinology

### Summary/Key Points

- Approximately 40% of people in the United States used complementary and alternative medicine (CAM) therapies in the past year.
- 17% of CAM therapies target otolaryngologic and rhinologic diagnoses, primarily allergic rhinitis, infectious rhinitis, and sinusitis.
- Nearly half of all CAM users do not communicate their use of these medications to their physicians.
- Perioperative risk of bleeding, anesthetic interactions, and other complications are possible with certain CAM medications.
- Preoperative evaluations must include a thorough history of any CAM use, and appropriate timing of discontinuation of these medications.

Complementary and alternative medicine (CAM) describes a broad category of practices and treatments for the prevention or treatment of disease outside of the realm of conventional medicine. CAM includes many types of interventions, from medications and supplements to physical therapies and procedures, and encompasses traditional Chinese medicine (herbal treatments and acupuncture therapy), homeopathy, naturopathy, herbal medicine, Ayurvedic medicine, mind-body medicine, chiropractic or osteopathic manipulations, and massage.

There is growing interest in and use of CAM, with CAM therapies for atopic conditions second only to treatments for back pain,[1] creating significant overlap of CAM with otolaryngology and rhinology. In 2007, 40% of adults in the United States had used at least 1 type of CAM in the previous year,[2] nearly doubling in the past 20 years, with current reports of 15% in Canada,[3] 25% in the United Kingdom,[4] and 50% use in Australia.[5] Fluctuation in the use of CAM over time seems to be influenced by cost, accessibility, failure of conventional medical therapies, cultural influences, and portrayal of CAM in the media.[6]

Popular conceptions of CAM as natural or harmless may also contribute to underreporting of CAM use, with patients often perceiving CAM or herbal medications to be a separate entity from traditional medications. Between 40% and 70% of patients

The authors have nothing to disclose.

[a] Department of Surgery, Division of Otolaryngology, University of Connecticut School of Medicine, 263 Farmington Avenue, Farmington, CT 06030, USA
[b] Connecticut Sinus Institute, 21 South Road, Suite 112, Farmington, CT 06032, USA
* Corresponding author. Connecticut Sinus Institute, 21 South Road, Suite 112, Farmington, CT 06032.
E-mail address: sbrown@prohealthmd.com

do not discuss their herbal medications, supplements, or other CAM therapeutics with their physicians,[4,7,8] and may not realize that a specific therapy is categorized as CAM. Conflicting pharmacodynamics, direct effects, and side effects of these undisclosed medications may lead to herb-drug interactions and adverse effects. Direct questioning from physicians is the strongest factor correlated with improved disclosure of CAM therapies,[3] but many physicians are unaware of the prevalence of CAM or its potential uses and risks. Evidence-based data on CAM therapies are often limited in depth or quality, or simply difficult to find in readily available publications. The rapid increase of CAM-related publications[3–6,8–19] in otolaryngology in the past decade highlights a growing awareness of CAM in the specialty, as well as the continuing need for data evaluating of the efficacy and safety of these therapies.

## RHINOLOGY AND COMPLEMENTARY MEDICINE

CAM is used for otolaryngology-specific ailments including allergic rhinitis, sinusitis, facial headache, tinnitus, and vertigo, with 17% of CAM use related to otolaryngologic diagnoses.[6] Sinusitis (chronic, acute, and allergic) and rhinitis (allergic, vasomotor, and infectious) are common targets of CAM in rhinology, with up to 30% of patients with chronic rhinosinusitis (CRS) using alternative herbal therapy before seeking conventional medical intervention.[12] Although conventional treatments for rhinitis or sinusitis typically include decongestants, antihistamines, steroids, antibiotics, and surgery, described CAM treatment options for rhinologic disease vary widely. Common types of CAM rhinologic treatments include nutritional supplements, herbal medications, homeopathy (use of diluted extracts), acupuncture (use of needles to affect physiologic function), aromatherapy, chiropractic (treatment by spinal manipulation), osteopathy (treatment of underlying mechanical disorders), and phototherapy (treatment with light). Details of many available CAM treatments are described in **Table 1**, including their active compounds, possible indications, and methods of use, as well as significant drug interactions and adverse effects.

### Nutritional Supplements

Ascorbic acid, or vitamin C, is used to treat infectious rhinitis (common cold) with 1 to 3 g by mouth daily, and allergic rhinitis as an intranasal topical medication. It seems to inhibit histamine secretion by lymphocytes, showing an inverse correlation of plasma ascorbic acid levels with histamine

levels.[20] Although ascorbic acid does not prevent acute viral rhinitis from the common cold, it may shorten the disease course by 1 to 1.5 days. Comparisons of intranasal ascorbic acid with placebo in allergic rhinitis have shown decreased nasal secretions, congestion, and edema in subjects treated with ascorbic acid solution.[20] Potential severe side effects include kidney stones, severe diarrhea, delayed healing, increased iron absorption in blood-iron disorders (thalassemia, hemochromatosis), and worsening of sickle cell disease. Drug interactions include decreased effectiveness of HIV/AIDS medications amprenavir (Agenerase), nelfinavir (Viracept), ritonavir (Norvir), and saquinavir (Fortovase, Invirase). Large amounts of ascorbic acid may decrease the effectiveness of warfarin (Coumadin), requiring dose alterations, and can delay the metabolism of aspirin, potentiating its effects.

Capsaicin (8-methyl-$n$-vanillyl-6-nonenamide) is the natural product of chili peppers that produces their burning heat. It is assumed to block neuropeptides like substance P, affecting pain transmission. Substance P is also released from nasal mucosal cells, interacting with nasal innervation and increasing interleukin (IL)-6 production,[5] potentially at greater levels in allergic rhinitis. Capsaicin is used in topical applications for pain relief from muscular soreness and peripheral neuropathy, but investigations of capsaicin for treatment of allergic rhinitis to dust mites did not find any therapeutic effect.[5] No drug interactions are known, and systemic side effects are rare, but localized irritation can occur at the application site.

Fish oil contains eicosapentaenoic acid (EPA) and docosahexaenoic (DHA) acids, ω-3 fatty acids known to have antiinflammatory properties benefiting chronic inflammatory conditions. Similarly, cod liver oil, produced from the livers of cod, halibut, and other white fish, contains long-chain fatty acids as well as vitamin D, and shares the antiinflammatory properties of fish oil. Reduced intake of fish oil fatty acids may be associated with an increase in allergic rhinitis prevalence.[5] Limited benefit has been shown in other allergic diagnoses like asthma and atopic dermatitis. However, information on the effects of fish oil on allergic rhinitis is minimal or conflicting between studies, with one double-blinded, placebo-controlled study resulting in no significant differences, whereas cross-sectional studies may show reduced prevalence of allergic rhinitis with increased intake of fish oil.[5] The ω-3 fatty acids exert a dose-related increase on bleeding time, and should be used with caution in patients with bleeding disorders, on blood-thinning medications, or before elective

**Table 1**
**Herbs in treatment of nasal conditions**

| Medication | Use | Mechanism | Adverse Effects |
|---|---|---|---|
| **Supplements** | | | |
| Ascorbic acid | Acute infectious rhinitis | Inhibition of histamine release | Kidney stones, diarrhea, delayed healing, increased iron absorption in blood-iron disorders, worsening sickle cell disease |
| Capsaicin | Allergic rhinitis | Inhibition of substance P, IL-6 production | Localized irritation |
| Fish oil | Allergic rhinitis, antiinflammatory | Reduced production and effectiveness of prostaglandins | Dose-related increase on bleeding time, hypotension |
| Spirulina | Allergic rhinitis, antiinflammatory | Inhibition of histamine release, reduced IL-4, increased IgA production | Hepatotoxicity, heavy-metal contamination |
| **Herbal medications** | | | |
| Bromelain | Sinusitis, allergic rhinitis, mucolytic, antiinflammatory | Proteolysis, inhibition of prostaglandins | GI upset, rare allergic reaction |
| Garlic | Acute infectious rhinitis, cough, URI | Inhibition of prostaglandins, thromboxanes | Inhibition of cytochrome P450 metabolism, decreased platelet aggregation, potentiation of warfarin effect |
| Quercetin | Antiinflammatory, antihistamine | Antioxidant, inhibition of cyclooxygenase to reduce leukotrienes, prostaglandins; mast cell stabilizer | None reported |
| Butterbur | Allergic rhinitis | Inhibition of leukotriene and histamine synthesis, mast cell stabilizer | Raw butterbur extract alkaloids are hepatotoxic, carcinogenic; rare GI upset |
| Sinupret | Allergic rhinosinusitis | Mucolytic, antiviral, antiinflammatory | Kidney stones, allergic reactions, GI upset, numbness, dermatitis |
| Echinacea | Acute infectious rhinitis | Activation of T, B lymphocytes | GI upset, headache, muscular ache, dizziness; hepatotoxicity with prolonged use |
| Esberitox | Acute sinusitis | Immune stimulation | Rash, itching, facial swelling, vertigo, hypotension |
| Cineole | Acute rhinosinusitis | Antiinflammatory, increased ciliary movement | Reflux, headache, nausea |

*(continued on next page)*

**Table 1**
*(continued)*

| Medication | Use | Mechanism | Adverse Effects |
|---|---|---|---|
| Angelica | URI, allergic rhinitis, cough, expectorant | Inhibition of prostaglandin E2 | Photosensitivity |
| Ephedra | Nasal congestion | Increased activity of noradrenaline on adrenergic receptors | Tachycardia, palpitations, hallucinations, hypertension, paranoia |
| Licorice root | Allergic rhinitis | Antiinflammatory, inhibition of 11-β-hydroxysteroid dehydrogenase, complement pathway | Hypokalemia, muscle ache, numbness, pseudoaldosteronism |
| *N*-Acetylcysteine | Sinusitis, mucolytic | Cleavage of disulfide bonds in mucoprotein | Rare GI upset |
| Shi-bi-lin | Allergic rhinitis, sneezing, nasal itching | Inhibition of IL-4 and TNF-α | None reported |
| Xiao-qing-long-tang | Infectious rhinitis, allergic rhinitis | Inhibition of histamine signaling, IL-4 and IL-5 | None reported |

*Abbreviations:* Ig, immunoglobulin; IL, interleukin; GI, gastrointestinal; TNF, tumor necrosis factor; URI, upper respiratory infection.

surgery. Fish oil can decrease blood pressure and increase the effect of hypertensive medications, leading to hypotension.

Spirulina is dried filamentous cyanobacteria from blue-green algae *Arthospira platensis* and is high in protein, vitamin B12 and provitamin A (β-carotenes), and minerals like iron. It is known to have antiinflammatory effects through inhibition of histamine release from mast cells, and high doses of spirulina significantly reduce IL-4 in the immunoglobulin (Ig)-E–mediated allergy pathway, and enhance IgA production. One randomized-control trial confirmed the decrease in IL-4 and improvement in nasal symptom scores in patients with allergic rhinitis after 6 months of spirulina dosing.[13] Hepatotoxicity and reactions from heavy-metal contamination have been reported but no drug interactions are known.

## Herbal Medications

Bromelain is a stem and fruit extract from pineapple (*Ananas comosus*) containing a proteolytic enzyme complex that has been used as a mucolytic and antiinflammatory. Use of bromelain has been shown to thin nasal mucus secretions, and is an effective mucolytic for the respiratory tract. Proteolysis at sites of inflammation also seems to inhibit the production proinflammatory prostaglandins like prostaglandin E1. A recent study from 2005 found statistically faster symptomatic recovery from sinusitis with bromelain compared with placebo.[20] Possible side effects are gastrointestinal upset and rare allergic reactions, with possible overlap with allergies to pineapple, wheat, celery, papain, carrot, fennel, cypress pollen, or grass pollen. Oral dosing of bromelain is typically 500 to 1000 mg/d or up to 2000 mg.

Garlic (*Allium sativum*) is often used for treatment of cough, viral upper respiratory infections, and rhinitis by oral dosing or direct nasal topical application. Potential adverse effects include rare allergic reactions, hypoglycemia, and prolonged bleeding time. Garlic also influences the cytochrome P450 system, potentiating the anticoagulant effect of warfarin.[1] Alterations of pharmacokinetics may also interfere with paracetamol and chlorpropamide, resulting in hypoglycemia, or ampicillin with increased minimal inhibitory concentration reported. Garlic is associated with decreased platelet aggregation within 5 days of oral dosing in a dose-dependent manner, with the possible mechanism being from inhibition of epinephrine-induced platelet aggregation.[7] Irreversible platelet effects from ajolene, another active compound in garlic, can increase the effects of other platelet inhibitors.[4] Discontinuing garlic intake 1 week before elective surgery is suggested. Although few published reports of bleeding complications have been connected to garlic, there are definitive reports of increased international normalized ratios (INRs) and prothrombin times with coinciding garlic and coumadin dosing.

Quercetin (3,3',4',5-7-pentahydroxyflavone) is a plant-derived flavonoid found in fruits, vegetables, leaves, and grains and exhibits in vitro antiinflammatory activity from antioxidant properties and inhibition of inflammatory enzymes (cyclooxygenase and lipooxygenase, regulators of leukotrienes and prostaglandins). In addition,, quercetin is able to stabilize mast cells to inhibit the release of histamine, even after IgE activation, and provides a clinical function similar to cromolyn sodium, although no definitive evidence of effect has been shown in clinical trials. Oral dosing with 400 to 500 mg 3 times daily is common. No side effects have been reported, but quercetin may lessen the effects of quinolone antibiotics, and these should not be taken simultaneously.

Butterbur (Petsites hybridus) is an extract from the leaves and roots of the butterbur shrub, and contains the active ingredient sesquiterpenes (petasins) that may inhibit leukotriene, mast cell degranulation, and histamine synthesis. Butterbur has been shown to significantly reduce the symptoms of allergic rhinitis in randomized, double-blinded, placebo-controlled studies, and is similar in efficacy to cetirizine and fexofenadine, although other studies showed minimal effect.[5] Critical to the safety profile of butterbur is the processing of raw butterbur extract to remove pyrrolizidine alkaloids that are hepatotoxic and carcinogenic. Petasin is a processed butterbur extract with the alkaloids removed, and is approved for allergic rhinitis treatment in Switzerland. Adverse effects include only rare gastrointestinal complaints, although the mechanism of action and long-term effects are poorly understood.

Sinupret is a herbal preparation used widely in Europe, including extracts of elder flowers (Sambucus nigra), cowslip flowers (Primula veris), common sorrel (Rumex acetosa), European vervain (Verbena officinalis), and gentain (Gentaina lutea) root. Of 4 larger studies, 3 showed positive efficacy with antiviral, antiinflammatory, and mucus-thinning properties.[15] Reported adverse events included kidney stones, allergic reactions, gastrointestinal symptoms, numbness, and mild dermatitis. Sinupret interacts with therapeutic monoclonal antibodies (eg, adalimumab [Humira], bevacizumab [Avastin], infliximab [Remicade], and omalizumab [Xolair]), hypertensive medications, and immunosuppressants (tacrolimus, methotrexate, corticosteroids, mycophenolate, etanercept, and cyclosporine), and is not recommended in patients with hypertension, immunosuppression, or a history of kidney stones.[12]

Echinacea (Echinacea purpurea leaf and Echinacea pallida contain active components) is a herb shown to activate T and B lymphocytes invitro, leading to a potential application for viral rhinitis symptoms, and although several meta-analyses found positive effects, some studies have shown no effect.[11] As is true with many herbal medications, commercially available formulations of echinacea also vary widely in amount and type of active compounds, further complicating effective studies. Gastrointestinal upset, tongue numbness, headache, muscular aches, and dizziness can occur, and echinacea has been associated with hepatotoxicity after prolonged use beyond 8 weeks. Echinacea can delay the metabolism of caffeine, causing tachycardia and nervousness, and it increases the activity of the immune system, which could directly counteract any immune-suppressive medications.

Esberitox contains 3 herbs (Thuja occidentalis, Echinacea angustifolia, and Baptisia tinctoria) and acts as an immune stimulant. Studies comparing Esberitox with placebo and other CAM and traditional therapies showed good effect as an adjunct to doxycycline for treatment of acute sinusitis, with significant effect compared with placebo.[12] No drug interactions are known, but uncommon side effects like rashes, itching, facial swelling, vertigo, and hypotension have been described.

Stinging nettle (Urtica doica) is used for the treatment of allergic rhinitis, but double-blind randomized studies have shown no, or only subjective, benefit.[1]

Myrtol is a herbal extract with components from Pinus spp (pine), Citrus aurantifolia (lime), and Eucalyptus globulus. Some effect compared with placebo has been shown, with symptom reduction similar to other herbal therapies but insufficient data to show significance.[12] Possible adverse effects included gastrointestinal disturbance, facial swelling and allergic reactions, and taste disturbances.

Cineole (eucalyptol or 1,8-cineole) is an active molecule extracted from eucalyptus oil for use in medications, with possible antiinflammatory benefits, as well as effect on ciliary movement with increased beat frequency.[15] It has been shown to augment the effectiveness of nasal decongestants for the treatment of acute rhinosinusitis compared with placebo,[12] particularly when dosed early in the course of an infection. Mild side effects such as reflux, headache, and nausea have been reported from Cineole, but possible serious side effects from pure eucalyptus oil are well known. Undiluted eucalyptus oil is potentially very toxic, through both oral and topical dosing, and 3.5 mL of undiluted oil can be fatal. Signs of eucalyptus poisoning are dizziness, weakness, mydriasis, shortness of breath, and abdominal pain or burning.

Angelica (*Angelica archangelica*) or danngui is commonly used for upper respiratory illnesses, allergies, and coughs as an expectorant. Some inhibitory effect on prostaglandin E2 is seen, as well as inhibition of the cytochrome P450 pathway, although the mechanism of action is not known.[1] Side effects like photosensitivity may occur.

Ephedra (*Ephedra sinica*) or ma huang contains high levels of ephedrine, and is often used for asthma, bronchitis, and nasal congestion, and as a weight loss aid and stimulant. The action of ephedrine can also lead to many serious side effects like tachycardia, palpitations, hallucinations, hypertension, paranoia, and potentially death, leading to a ban of ephedra in the United States.[21] There are multiple interactions with drugs like glycosides and halothane causing arrhythmias and potentiation of monoamine oxidase inhibitors (MAOIs).

Licorice root (*Glycyrrhiza glabra*) is used in the treatment of allergic rhinitis, conjunctivitis, and bronchitis as an antiinflammatory, and antiviral activity has been noted on in vitro studies. Licorice is known to inhibit 11-β-hydroxysteroid dehydrogenase and the classic complement pathway, and side effects can include hypokalemia, muscle pain, extremity numbness, and pseudoaldosteronism, which leads to hypertension, headaches, and cardiac events.[7] Risk for adverse events is higher with large doses, but can occur at low doses as well. Licorice also interferes with angiotensin-converting enzyme (ACE)–inhibitors, diuretics, corticosteroids, insulin and other diabetic drugs, MAOIs, oral contraceptives, and digoxin, where licorice can dangerously increase the toxicity of digoxin.

*N*-acetylcysteine (NAC) is used in the treatment of sinusitis primarily for its mucolytic properties, achieved through cleavage of disulfide bonds in mucoproteins by its sulfhydryl group resulting in less-viscous mucus.[20] No serious side effects are known, but occasional gastrointestinal disturbances can occur. Adult dose is 600 to 1500 mg a day split into 8-hourly doses.

## Ayurvedic Medicine

Ayurvedic medicine (from the Sanskrit *ayur* meaning life, and *veda* meaning science) is a traditional medical ideology originating in India with the goal of balancing the body, mind, and spirit through herbal medications, massage, and specific diets. More than 600 multiherb formulas and 250 single-herb medications are included in the Ayurvedic repertoire, including Aller-7 and Tinofend, which have been described for use in allergic rhinitis.

Aller-7 is a formulation of herbal extracts including quercetin, stinging nettles, methylsulfonylmethane, turmeric, feverfew, ginger, and vitamin C. It has shown some improvement in allergic rhinitis symptoms by possibly reducing inflammation.[5]

Tinofend is a herbal tablet of *Tinospora cordifolia* that has shown efficacy compared with placebo; however, no studies have comprehensive data supporting the use of Aller-7 or Tinofend for allergic rhinitis.

## Chinese traditional medicine

Shi-bi-lin is a Chinese herbal medication used for sneezing and nasal itching associated with allergic rhinitis, and is thought to act by inhibiting release of IL-4 and tumor necrosis factor (TNF)–α.[5] Animal trials have shown efficacy and decreased eosinophil infiltration. Human safety trials are in progress, with similar improvement in symptoms to placebo, but a prolonged effect.

Xiao-qing-long-tang (Sho-seiryu-to in Japanese, or TJ-19) consists of extracts from 8 herbs, including ephedra. It is used for infectious rhinitis, asthma, and allergic rhinitis, and shows inhibition of histamine signaling and IL-4 and IL-5 expression in rat models.[5]

Acupuncture is commonly used for CRS in Chinese traditional medicine, and 5% of adults in the United States have tried acupuncture for CRS. These techniques are thought to reduce inflammation and lead to desensitization to underlying allergy.[21] One study evaluating efficacy of acupuncture showed a nonsignificant improvement in CRS symptoms over several weeks of acupuncture therapy compared with conventional treatment.[22]

## Other therapies

Homeopathy involves treatment with stimulating active agents dosed at ultradiluted amounts based on an individual's symptomatic response.[5] Studies of homeopathic treatments vary in evidence-based reports of benefit, and occasionally have been shown to worsen symptoms.

Phototherapy uses topical illumination with specific wavelengths of light to prompt an immunosuppressive response. This technique reduces antigen presentation by dendritic cells and inhibits

**Table 2**
Recommendations and implications of natural product use as related to preoperative concerns

| Natural Product | Evidence-based Recommendations: Discontinuation of Natural Products Before Surgery (wk) | Perioperative Concerns |
|---|---|---|
| Fish oil | 2–3[25] | Perioperative bleeding[25,26] Hypotension[26] |
| Glucosamine | 2–3[25] | Hypoglycemia[25,27] |
| Garlic | 1[25,28] At least 2[29,30] | Perioperative bleeding[25–29,31–34] Hypotension[25–28,31] |
| Flax seed | No specific recommendations | Perioperative bleeding[35] |
| Coenzyme Q-10 (ubiquinone) | No specific recommendations | Hypotension[26] Cardiac effects[26] Perioperative bleeding effects[34] |
| Saw palmetto | 2–3[25] | Perioperative bleeding[25,31] Tachycardia[31] Angina[31] Water/electrolyte disturbances[27] |
| Ginseng | At least 1[25,32] At least 2[29] | Hypoglycemia[25,27,28,31–33] Hypertension[25,28,31,32] Perioperative bleeding[25–27,29,31–34] Tachycardia[31,32] Water/electrolyte disturbances[27] Prolongation of anesthetic effects[27] |
| Chondroitin | 2–3[25] | Perioperative bleeding[25,27] |
| Milk thistle | 2–3[25] | Volume depletion[25] |
| Green tea | No specific recommendations | Perioperative bleeding[34,35] Cardiovascular side effects[34,35] Water/electrolyte disturbances[27] |

*Data from* King A, Russett F, Generali J, et al. Evaluation and implications of natural product use in preoperative patients: a retrospective review. BMC Complement Altern Med 2009;9(1):38.

proinflammatory factors, decreasing nasal symptom scores and levels of IL-5 and eosinophils.[5]

Nasosympatico treatment stimulates and medicates the nasal mucosa directly by applying essential oils directly to the sinus ostia on soft cotton swabs.

Nasal saline irrigation provides benefits of mechanical clearing of mucus, thinner mucus, and improved mucociliary clearance at minimal cost or risk to the patient. Isotonic and hypertonic saline nasal rinses have been shown to significantly improve the symptoms of rhinosinusitis.[19] Isotonic saline rinses significantly increased mucociliary clearance time in acute rhinosinusitis; however, hypertonic saline rinses improved clearance time only in patients with chronic sinusitis.[23]

## SUMMARY OF CAM USE IN RHINOLOGY MEDICINE AND SURGERY

Considering the prevalence of CAM use generally and within rhinology, and the potential for side effects and drug-drug interactions,[7,24] it is critical for physicians to have a broad knowledge of CAM therapeutics and their benefits and pitfalls. Consistently asking patients about CAM use, and tracking CAM medications and dosing in the same way as conventional medications, provides clinicians with the knowledge they need to thoroughly monitor adverse effects and medication conflicts.

From the surgical perspective, the possibility of a CAM therapy's impact on bleeding can be critical during the preoperative and perioperative period. Safety profiles and mechanisms for CAM therapies are often poorly understood because of a paucity of in-depth research. This situation becomes even more critical during surgery when factoring in the higher risk of exposure to multiple complex drugs and the systemic stress of surgery. The American Society of Anesthesiologists (ASA) recently released recommendations for patients to discontinue all herbal medications 2 to 4 weeks before surgery. CAM medications that alter platelet function or aggregation, affect the coagulation cascade, or otherwise affect coagulation include ascorbic acid, fish oil, vitamin E, garlic, echinacea, ginseng, ginger, and ginkgo biloba **(Table 2)**.[8,36] Also important is the impact of any CAM therapies on wound healing, their drug-drug interactions with postoperative analgesics or antibiotics, anesthetic agents, and other perioperative medications. Within the physician-patient relationship, it is also important to communicate clearly to the patient that CAM therapies are drugs just as conventional medicines are, and reporting CAM medication use, changes, or problems is important. Continuing research is needed to develop a thorough, evidence-based library of CAM data with randomized-controlled trials, and improving standardization of the CAM pharmaceuticals industry will better ensure consistency of a CAM medication concentration and effect.

# REFERENCES

1. Bielory L. Complementary and alternative interventions in asthma, allergy, and immunology. Ann Allergy Asthma Immunol 2004;93(2 Suppl 1):S45–54.
2. Neiberg RH, Aickin M, Grzywacz JG, et al. Occurrence and co-occurrence of types of complementary and alternative medicine use by age, gender, ethnicity, and education among adults in the United States: the 2002 National Health Interview Survey (NHIS). J Altern Complement Med 2011;17(4):363–70.
3. Rotenberg BW, Bertens KA. Use of complementary and alternative medical therapies for chronic rhinosinusitis: a Canadian perspective. J Otolaryngol Head Neck Surg 2010;39(5):586–93.
4. Shakeel M, Trinidade A, Ah-See KW. Complementary and alternative medicine use by otolaryngology patients: a paradigm for practitioners in all surgical specialties. Eur Arch Otorhinolaryngol 2010;267(6):961–71.
5. Man LX. Complementary and alternative medicine for allergic rhinitis. Curr Opin Otolaryngol Head Neck Surg 2009;17(3):226–31.
6. Shakeel M, Trinidade A, Jehan S, et al. The use of complementary and alternative medicine by patients attending a general otolaryngology clinic: can we afford to ignore it? Am J Otolaryngol 2010; 31(4):252–60.
7. Miller LG. Herbal medicinals: selected clinical considerations focusing on known or potential drug-herb interactions. Arch Intern Med 1998; 158(20):2200–11.
8. Shakeel M, Newton JR, Ah-See KW. Complementary and alternative medicine use among patients undergoing otolaryngologic surgery. J Otolaryngol Head Neck Surg 2009;38(3):355–61.
9. Raghavan U, Jones NS. Complementary and alternative therapy for nasal conditions. J Laryngol Otol 2000;114(12):919–24.
10. Krouse JH, Krouse HJ. Patient use of traditional and complementary therapies in treating rhinosinusitis before consulting an otolaryngologist. Laryngoscope 1999;109(8):1223–7.
11. Asher BF, Seidman M, Snyderman C. Complementary and alternative medicine in otolaryngology. Laryngoscope 2001;111(8):1383–9.
12. Guo R, Canter PH, Ernst E. Herbal medicines for the treatment of rhinosinusitis: a systematic review. Otolaryngol Head Neck Surg 2006;135(4):496–506.
13. Karkos PD, Leong SC, Arya AK, et al. "Complementary ENT": a systematic review of commonly used supplements. J Laryngol Otol 2007;121(8): 779–82.
14. Shakeel M, Little SA, Bruce J, et al. Use of complementary and alternative medicine in pediatric otolaryngology patients attending a tertiary hospital in the UK. Int J Pediatr Otorhinolaryngol 2007;71(11):1725–30.
15. Tesche S, Metternich F, Sonnemann U, et al. The value of herbal medicines in the treatment of acute non-purulent rhinosinusitis. Results of a double-blind, randomised, controlled trial. Eur Arch Otorhinolaryngol 2008;265(11):1355–9.
16. Shakeel M, Newton JR, Bruce J, et al. Use of complementary and alternative medicine by patients attending a head and neck oncology clinic. J Laryngol Otol 2008;122(12):1360–4.
17. Lim CM, Ng A, Loh KS. Use of complementary and alternative medicine in head and neck cancer patients. J Laryngol Otol 2010;124(5):529–32.
18. Vyas T, Hart RD, Trites JR, et al. Complementary and alternative medicine use in patients presenting to a head and neck oncology clinic. Head Neck 2010;32(6):793–9.
19. Ural A, Oktemer TK, Kizil Y, et al. Impact of isotonic and hypertonic saline solutions on mucociliary activity in various nasal pathologies: clinical study. J Laryngol Otol 2009;123:517–21.
20. Helms S, Miller A. Natural treatment of chronic rhinosinusitis. Altern Med Rev 2006;11(3):196–207.
21. Zijlstra FJ, van den Berg-de Lange I, Huygen FJ, et al. Anti-inflammatory actions of acupuncture. Mediators Inflamm 2003;12(2):59–69.
22. Rössberg E, Larsson PG, Birkeflet O, et al. Comparison of traditional Chinese acupuncture, minimal acupuncture at non-acupoints and conventional

treatment for chronic sinusitis. Complement Ther Med 2005;13(1):4–10.

23. Blanc PD, Trupin L, Earnest G, et al. Alternative therapies among adults with a reported diagnosis of asthma or rhinosinusitis : data from a population-based survey. Chest 2001;120(5):1461–7.

24. Ernst E. Harmless herbs? a review of the recent literature. Am J Med 1998;104(2):170–8.

25. Heller J, Gabbay JS, Ghadjar K, et al. Top-10 list of herbal and supplemental medicines used by cosmetic patients: what the plastic surgeon needs to know. Plast Reconstr Surg 2006;117:436–45.

26. Wren KR, Kimbrall S, Norred CL. Use of complementary and alternative medications by surgical patients. J Perianesth Nurs 2002;17:170–7.

27. Cheng B, Hung CT, Chiu W. Herbal medicine and anesthesia. Hong Kong Med J 2002;8:123–30.

28. Hodges P, Kam P. The peri-operative implications of herbal medicines. Anaesthesia 2002;57:889–99.

29. Pass S, Simpson R. Discontinuation and reinstitution of medications during the perioperative period. Am J Health Syst Pharm 2004;61:899–914.

30. Mikail C, Hearney E, Nemesure B. Increasing physician awareness of the common uses and contraindication of herbal medicines: utility of a case-based tutorial for residents. J Altern Complement Med 2003;9:571–6.

31. Tessier D, Bash D. A surgeon's guide to herbal supplements. J Surg Res 2003;114:30–6.

32. Mackichan C, Ruthman J. Herbal product use and preoperative patients. AORN J 2004;79:948–59.

33. Ang-Lee M, Moss J, Yuan C. Herbal medicines and perioperative care. JAMA 2001;286:208–16.

34. Heck A, DeWitt BA, Lukes AL. Potential interactions between alternative therapies and warfarin. Am J Health Syst Pharm 2000;57:1221–7.

35. Kumar N, Allen K, Bell H. Perioperative herbal supplement use in cancer patients: potential implications and recommendations for presurgical screening. Cancer Control 2005;12:149–57.

36. King A, Russett F, Generali J, et al. Evaluation and implications of natural product use in preoperative patients: a retrospective review. BMC Complement Altern Med 2009;9(1):38.

# Sinonasal Problems and Reflux

Todd A. Loehrl, MD

## KEYWORDS

- Reflux • GER • Rhinosinusitis • Evidence levels
- Pediatric treatment outcomes • Adult treatment outcomes

---

**Key Points**

- Relationship between reflux and rhinosinusitis still poorly defined.
- Reflux may be the cause of some symptoms attributed to rhinosinusitis (eg, postnasal drip).
- Consider reflux as a factor in patients with refractory sinonasal inflammatory disease.

---

The gastrointestinal tract was implicated in the pathogenesis of chronic sinusitis more than 50 years ago when Holmes and colleagues[1] proposed a connection between sinonasal disease and gastric hypersecretion. However, it has only been in the last few years that clinicians' awareness of gastroesophageal reflux (GER) as a potential exacerbating factor of upper airway inflammatory disease has increased. Thus far, most studies evaluating the association have been retrospective and a scientifically valid relationship remains elusive.

To solidify the association between GER and chronic rhinosinusitis (CRS), 3 criteria should be met:

1. Patients with CRS should have a higher prevalence of GER than patients without CRS.
2. The pathophysiologic mechanisms between GER and CRS should help explain how the disease processes interact.
3. If GER is a contributing factor to CRS, then GER treatment should improve or resolve CRS in most patients.

This article reviews the literature regarding these criteria.

## PREVALENCE OF GER IN PATIENTS WITH CRS

DiBaise and colleagues[2] showed a high prevalence of GER in patients with CRS. They found that 78% of patients with CRS had GER based on 24-hour esophageal pH monitoring (pH<4.0 more than 9.2% of total time at the distal site or more than 3.3% of total time at the proximal site). Furthermore, results from a large case-control epidemiologic study showed that adults with complicated GER were more likely to have sinusitis (odds ratio, 1.60; 95% confidence interval [CI], 1.51–1.70) than were controls.[3] Pincus and colleagues[4] also found reflux in 25 of 30 patients with CRS. These 25 patients were placed on proton pump inhibitor therapy and were reevaluated 1 month later, at which point 14 of 15 evaluable patients reported improvement in their symptoms, including 7 who had almost/complete resolution. However, several methodological problems limit interpretation of the study including, but not limited to, the short follow-up, lack of a control group, the potential for recall bias, as well as limited documentation of CRS disease severity. Furthermore, Onerci and colleagues,[5] using a nasal lavage pepsin assay and 24-hour dual-probe monitoring, found that 88% of patients with CRS had pharyngeal acid reflux compared with 55% of controls. The investigators acknowledged the higher incidence (55%) of reflux in the control group than previously reported. The investigators attributed this finding to the nutritional habits of the Turkish population, although they did not elaborate on the nature of the potential causative nutritional habits.

---

Department of Otolaryngology and Communication Sciences, Zablocki VA Medical Center, Medical College of Wisconsin, 5000 West National Avenue, Milwaukee, WI 53202, 53214, USA
*E-mail address:* tloehrl@mcw.edu

Facial Plast Surg Clin N Am 20 (2012) 83–86
doi:10.1016/j.fsc.2011.10.009
1064-7406/12/$ – see front matter Published by Elsevier Inc

## Studies on GER and Refractory CRS

A few studies have specifically investigated medically and surgically refractory CRS.

Ulualp and colleagues[6] also showed a significantly higher prevalence of GER in patients with CRS unresponsive to conventional therapy compared with normal controls ($P<.05$), and postulated that GER may contribute to the pathogenesis of CRS in some adult patients.

Chambers and colleagues[7] found that the presence of GER was a predictor of poor symptomatic outcome after sinus surgery in adults.

Similarly, Delgaudio,[8] using a specially designed pH probe, showed increased reflux at the nasopharynx, upper esophageal sphincter, and distal esophagus in patients with medically and surgically refractory rhinosinusitis compared with controls. He concluded that it is likely that reflux is an important causative factor of refractory CRS in adults. Although his study does show an association, causation is far from clear given from the information provided. In an unpublished study, our group studied 22 patients with medically and surgically refractory rhinosinusitis. All subjects underwent comprehensive testing for extraesophageal reflux (EER) including 24-hour pharyngeal pH probe, aerosolized nasopharyngeal pH testing, and nasopharyngeal tissue biopsy for pepsin analysis. In addition, the last 5 subjects underwent nasal secretion analysis for pepsin. A control group of healthy subjects underwent the same nasal secretion pepsin analysis. The pharyngeal pH probe results were positive in 19 of 20 (95%), whereas the DeMeester score was positive in 9 of 19 (47%). The nasopharyngeal pH probe data were available in 17 of 20 patients and correlated poorly with the pharyngeal pH probe testing. In all 20 subjects, nasopharyngeal tissue biopsies were negative for pepsin. However, the 5 subjects who underwent nasal pepsin analysis were all pepsin positive, whereas 5 healthy controls nasal lavages were negative for pepsin. Thus this study supports an association of EER with medically and surgically refractory CRS.

The finding of pepsin in nasal aspirates suggests that direct contact of the refluxate with the paranasal sinus mucosa may play a role in the pathophysiology of CRS in this patient population. In addition, evaluation for pepsin in nasal fluid is a viable method for determining the presence of refluxate in the nose and paranasal sinuses (Loehrl TA and colleagues Triological Thesis *Reflux and Refractory Chronic Rhinosinusitis*. September, 2010).

In children, several investigators have suggested a relationship between GER and CRS.[9–13] Contencin and Narcy[9] initially showed a possible relationship between GER and chronic upper airway inflammation in the pediatric population. Subsequent studies, both retrospective[11,12] and prospective,[10] have shown a high prevalence of GER (especially pharyngeal reflux) in children with CRS, providing further evidence in support of the relationship. These studies are all retrospective and lack control groups.

## POSSIBLE PATHOPHYSIOLOGIC MECHANISMS BETWEEN REFLUX AND CRS

The mechanism(s) by which reflux affects the sinonasal cavity remains unclear, but 3 mechanisms have been proposed:

1. Refluxate effect on the mucosa
2. Vagally mediated neurogenic mechanism(s)
3. *Helicobacter pylori.*

### Refluxate Effect on Mucosa

The first proposed mechanism is that the refluxate has a direct effect on the mucosa, resulting in an inflammatory response with edema and impaired mucociliary clearance. These events result in sinus ostial obstruction and infection. In children, reflux to the nasopharynx has been shown using 24-hour pH probe studies.[9,10] In infants and children with previously documented reflux, Contencin and Narcy[9] showed that, when a 2-site pH probe was placed with one site in the esophagus and the other in the hypopharynx, refluxate frequently extended above the cricopharyngeus. Phipps and colleagues[10] showed that 63% of patients with CRS showed GER, which is considerably more than the prevalence in a normal healthy population. Furthermore, 32% of these patients showed nasopharyngeal reflux. In addition, as noted earlier, in an unpublished study, our group showed pepsin in nasal secretions in all 5 patients with medically/surgically refractory rhinosinusitis, whereas none of the healthy controls had evidence of pepsin in their nasal secretions.

### Neurogenic Mechanism

The second theory revolves around a vagally mediated neurogenic mechanism. This mechanism may involve dysfunction of the autonomic nervous system, resulting in sinonasal edema and secondary ostial obstruction. This disorder has been shown in the lower airway by Lodi and colleagues[14] and Harding and colleagues.[15] They found that patients with asthma and GER disease have exaggerated vagal responsiveness, compared with age-matched controls. Dysfunction of the autonomic nervous system was shown by Loehrl and colleagues[16] in patients with chronic upper airway inflammation. They found that these patients, compared with a group of age-matched and sex-matched controls, have significant ($P = .02$) autonomic nervous system dysfunction characterized by adrenergic hypofunction. In addition, it was noted that patients with documented extraesophageal reflux and vasomotor rhinitis had statistically significant evidence of more adrenergic hypofunction than those with vasomotor rhinitis alone.

## H pylori

The third possible mechanism involves the potential role of H pylori in CRS. H pylori is a microaerophilic gram-negative spiral organism that has been shown to play a large role in stomach ulcers and gastritis.[17,18] It has also been shown in human dental plaque,[19] oral lesions[20] and saliva.[21] Ozdek and colleagues[22] used polymerase chain reaction to detect H pylori in 4 of 12 patients with CRS, whereas it was not detected in any patient without CRS. In 3 of the 4 patients in whom H pylori was detected, the patients had GER-related complaints. However, it remains unknown whether H pylori is a causative agent for CRS or whether it results from CRS.

## TREATMENT OUTCOMES FOR CRS WITH REFLUX TREATMENT

Regarding GER treatment improving or resolving CRS in most patients if it is a true contributing factor, the outcome of reflux therapy in pediatric chronic rhinosinusitis is more convincing than in adults, although well-designed studies are lacking. Bothwell and colleagues[11] found that, in children with medically refractory CRS, 89% experienced relief of their symptoms with reflux therapy and were able to avoid sinus surgery. They concluded that gastronasal reflux should be evaluated and treated before sinus surgery. Similarly, Phipps and colleagues[10] found that upper airway symptoms improved in 79% of patients with CRS and GER after reflux treatment. In a retrospective review of adults with GER and chronic refractory rhinosinusitis, DiBaise and colleagues[2] found that 67% of patients noted improvement in sinus symptoms after undergoing therapy for GER. In addition, the patients with abnormal 24-hour pH testing tended to have a more dramatic response to therapy. In a follow-up prospective study, modest improvement in sinus symptoms was found after treatment with twice-a-day proton pump inhibitors for 3 months. Despite these improvements, complete symptom resolution occurred infrequently. In addition, they found that pH test results did not predict symptomatic outcome.[23]

There are a few possible reasons for the incomplete response to therapy in the studies mentioned earlier:

- The duration of treatment was only 3 months, whereas the current recommendations are for twice-a-day dosing of proton pump inhibitors for a minimum of 6 months.[24]
- Amin and colleagues[25] documented that 44% of patients on twice-a-day proton pump inhibitor dosing still have abnormal levels of acid exposure, based on dual-probe pH testing.
- Pepsin may play a role in addition to the role traditionally attributed to acid, and has been documented to contribute to mucosal injury as much or more than acid exposure.[26]
- Previous studies suggested that pepsin activity declines at pH 4 to 5, but more recent tests have shown that pH 7 does not completely denature pepsin.[27]

Although there are few data supporting the efficacy of EER treatment in this patient population, medical and surgical therapy can be selectively considered. In addition to acid suppression, other nonsurgical therapeutic options are being developed, such as mucosal pepsin receptor antagonists.[28] In addition, a promising liquid alginate preparation is available in Europe, but not yet in the United States.[29] Little evidence exists for surgical therapy. However, in patients with well-documented GER disease and refractory airway disease, Nissen fundoplication may be an alternative. Further investigation needs to be performed regarding the role of Nissen fundoplication in patients with EER alone.

## SUMMARY OF THE ROLE OF GER IN CRS

It is possible that GER plays a role in some patients with CRS, based on the increased prevalence of GER in patients with CRS, the possible pathophysiologic mechanisms linking the disorders, and the response to therapy noted. However, more work needs to be done to solidify the relationship, especially with regard to the pathophysiology linking CRS and GER, as well as the reasons for a lack of therapeutic response in some patients.

## REFERENCES

1. Holmes TH, Goodell H, Wolf S, et al. The nose: an experimental study of reactions within the nose in human subjects during various life experiences. Springfield (IL): Charles C Thomas; 1950. p. 1–54.
2. DiBaise JK, Huerter JV, Quigley E. Sinusitis and gastroesophageal reflux disease. Ann Intern Med 1998;129:1078.
3. el-Serag HB, Sonnenberg A. Comorbid occurrence of laryngeal or pulmonary disease with esophagitis in United States military veterans. Gastroenterology 1997;113:755–60.
4. Pincus RL, Kim HH, Silvers S, et al. A study of the link between gastric reflux and chronic sinusitis in adults. Ear Nose Throat J 2006;85(3):174–8.
5. Onerci M, Yücel OT, Sinici I, et al. Nasal pepsin assay and pH monitoring in chronic rhinosinusitis. Laryngoscope 2008;118:890–4.
6. Ulualp SO, Toohill RJ, Hoffmann R, et al. Possible relationship of gastroesophagopharyngeal acid reflux with pathogenesis of chronic sinusitis. Am J Rhinol 1999;13:197–202.
7. Chambers CW, Davis WE, Cook PR, et al. Long-term outcome analysis of functional endoscopic sinus surgery: correlation of symptoms with endoscopic examination findings and potential prognostic variables. Laryngoscope 1997;107:504–10.
8. Delgaudio JM. Direct nasopharyngeal reflux of gastric acid is a contributing factor in refractory chronic rhinosinusitis. Laryngoscope 2005;115(6): 946–57.
9. Contencin P, Narcy P. Nasopharyngeal pH monitoring in infants and children with chronic rhinopharyngitis. Int J Pediatr Otorhinolaryngol 1991;22:249–56.
10. Phipps CD, Wood WE, Gibson WS, et al. Gastroesophageal reflux contributing to chronic sinus disease in children. A prospective analysis. Arch Otolaryngol Head Neck Surg 1999;121:255–62.
11. Bothwell MR, Parsons DS, Tablot A, et al. Outcome of reflux therapy on pediatric chronic sinusitis. Otolaryngol Head Neck Surg 1999;121:255–62.
12. Halstead LA. Role of gastroesophageal reflux in pediatric upper airway disorders. Otolaryngol Head Neck Surg 1999;120:208–14.
13. Barbero GJ. Gastroesophageal reflux and upper airway disease: a commentary. Otolaryngol Clin North Am 1996;29:27–38.
14. Lodi U, Harding SM, Coghlan HC, et al. Autonomic regulation in asthmatics with gastroesophageal reflux. Chest 1997;111:65–70.
15. Harding SM, Guxxo MR, Maples RV, et al. Gastroesophageal reflux induced bronchoconstriction; vagolytic doses of atropine diminish airway responses to esophageal acid infusion [abstract]. Am J Respir Crit Care Med 1995;151:A589.
16. Loehrl TA, Smith TL, Darling RJ, et al. Autonomic dysfunction, vasomotor rhinitis, and extraesophageal manifestations of gastroesophageal reflux. Otolaryngol Head Neck Surg 2002;126:382–7.
17. Alper J. Ulcers as an infectious disease. Science 1993;260:159–60.
18. Lee A, Fox J, Hazell S. Pathogenicity of Helicobacter pylori: a perspective. Infect Immun 1993;61:1601–10.
19. Cammarota G, Tursi A, Montalto M, et al. Role of dental plaque in the transmission of Helicobacter pylori infection. J Clin Gastroenterol 1996;22: 174–7.
20. Mravak-Stipetic M, Gall-Troself K, Lukac J, et al. Detection of Helicobacter pylori in various oral lesions by nested polymerase chain reaction (PCR). J Oral Pathol Med 1998;27:1–3.
21. Li C, Musich PR, Has T, et al. High prevalence of Helicobacter pylori in saliva demonstrated by a novel PCR assay. J Clin Pathol 1995;48:662–6.
22. Ozdek A, Cirak MY, Samim E, et al. A possible role of Helicobacter pylori in chronic rhinosinusitis: a preliminary report. Laryngoscope 2003;113(4):679–82.
23. DiBaise JK, Olusola BF, Huerter JV, et al. Role GERD in chronic resistant sinusitis: a prospective, open label, pilot trial. Am J Gastroenterol 2002;97:843–50.
24. Postma GN, Johnson LF, Koufman JA. Treatment of laryngopharyngeal reflux. Ear Nose Throat J 2002; 81(9):24–6.
25. Amin MR, Postma GN, Johnson P, et al. Proton pump inhibitor resistance in the treatment of laryngopharyngeal reflux. Otolaryngol Head Neck Surg 2001; 125(4):374–8.
26. Tutian R, Maine I, Dgarwal A, et al. Non acid reflux in patients with chronic cough on acid suppressive therapy. Chest 2006;130:386–91.
27. Tasker A, Dettmar PW, Panetti M, et al. Is gastric reflux a cause of otitis media with effusion in children? Laryngoscope 2002;112(11):1930–4.
28. Sweet MP, Patti MG, Hoopes C, et al. Gastroesophageal reflux and aspiration in patients with advanced lung disease. Thorax 2009;64(2):167–73.
29. McGlashan JA, Johnstone LM, Strungala V, et al. The value of a liquid alginate suspension (Gaviscon Advance) in the management of laryngo-pharyngeal reflux. Eur Arch Otorhinolaryngol 2009;266(2): 243–51.

# Bacteriology and Antibiotic Resistance in Chronic Rhinosinusitis

R. Peter Manes, MD[a], Pete S. Batra, MD[b],*

## KEYWORDS

- Chronic rhinosinusitis • Bacteria • Microbiology of sinusitis
- Antibiotics • Bacterial resistance

---

### Key Points

- Through understanding of microbiology and drug resistance patterns of chronic rhinosinusitis is a requisite if the facial plastic surgeon contemplates concurrent rhinoplasty with FESS.
- The most common organisms assayed in acute rhinosinusitis include *Streptococcus pneumoniae*, *Moraxella catarrhalis*, and *Haemophilus influenzae*.
- The most common organisms cultured in chronic rhinosinusitis are *Staphylococcus aureus*, coagulase-negative *Staphylococcus*, and gram-negative rods.
- *S aureus* is the most common organism seen on chronic sinusitis; its presence during FESS is associated with postop *S aureus* infection and impaired mucosal healing.
- *Pseudomonas aeruginosa* is the most commonly cultured gram negative rod and can be a source of recalcitrance due to biofilm formation.
- *Strenotrophomonas maltophilia* is a multidrug resistant gram-negative microbe seen in patients with previous FESS and prior antimicrobial treatment.
- Judicious usage of antimicrobial therapy is recommended for infectious exacerbations of chronic rhinosinusitis, ideally with endoscopically-guided cultures.

---

## DILEMMAS IN CONCURRENT MANAGEMENT OF CHRONIC RHINOSINUSITIS IN THE RHINOPLASTY PATIENT

Chronic rhinosinusitis (CRS) ranks among the most common health problems in the United States.[1] The comprehensive management algorithm for CRS entails a variety of medical therapies, such as antibiotics, oral and/or nasal steroids, leukotriene antagonists, and saline irrigations, with functional endoscopic sinus surgery (FESS) being reserved for refractory cases. Current estimates suggest that the number of sinus surgeries performed in the United States approximates 250,000 annually.[2] In some instances, patients undergoing FESS may inquire about the possibility

---

Disclosures: P.S.B: consultant (Medtronic, LifeCell), research grants (ARS, Medtronic, MedInvent, Xoran). R.P.M: research grant (MedInvent).

[a] Section of Otolaryngology–Head and Neck Surgery, Department of Surgery, Yale University School of Medicine, 333 Cedar Street, PO Box 208041, New Haven, CT 06520, USA
[b] Comprehensive Skull Base Program, Department of Otolaryngology–Head and Neck Surgery, University of Texas Southwestern Medical Center, 5323 Harry Hines Boulevard, Dallas, TX 75390, USA
* Corresponding author.
E-mail address: pete.batra@utsouthwestern.edu

Facial Plast Surg Clin N Am 20 (2012) 87–91
doi:10.1016/j.fsc.2011.10.010

of concurrent reconstructive or cosmetic nasal surgery.

As our society becomes more concerned with appearance and plastic surgery procedures are more readily available and accepted, requests to combine elective aesthetic surgery with medical procedures will not be uncommon. Patients may view this as a means to decrease the number of operations performed for their overall care. Furthermore, the patient mindset may rationalize this approach with the thought that the surgeon "will be working on the nose anyway."

Diverging opinions exist on the concept of concurrent FESS and rhinoplasty.

### Arguments Against Concomitant FESS and Rhinoplasty

Some experts have advocated against these concomitant procedures for several important reasons.[3] Intranasal inflammation and intranasal incisions as a result of rhinoplasty greatly add to the postoperative discomfort and make any attempt at effective debridement exceedingly difficult. While the exact role of debridement is controversial, most rhinologists hold that timely debridement starting 1 week after surgery is imperative to decrease the risk of synechiae formation and to achieve optimally functioning postoperative sinonasal cavities. Furthermore, nasal manipulation for debridement in the early postoperative period may alter the delicate position of the nasal osteotomies and compromise the cosmetic and functional outcome. Another argument against concurrent rhinoplasty and FESS focuses on the possibility of infection, given that FESS often takes place in an infected sinonasal space. Osteotomies performed during rhinoplasty breach the periosteum, creating a potential route for the spread of infection. The use of synthetic graft material in rhinoplasty adds another complicating factor to the possible spread of infection, though avoidance of graft materials may worsen outcomes from rhinoplasty.

### Arguments for Concomitant FESS and Rhinoplasty

Conversely, others have argued that with appropriate and aggressive medical management of CRS, including preoperative, intraoperative, and postoperative antibiotic treatment, the risk of potential spread of infection to the nasal or facial tissues is greatly reduced.[4] Moreover, the patient is spared an additional anesthetic and postoperative recuperative period, perhaps resulting in cost savings in the long term. However, within that argument rests an important caveat: to provide appropriate medical management of CRS, one must understand both its bacteriology and antibiotic resistance patterns.

## BACTERIOLOGY OF RHINOSINUSITIS

Bacteria likely represent the main underlying cause of acute rhinosinusitis (ARS), with the most commonly identified bacteria being *Streptococcus pneumoniae*, *Moraxella catarrhalis*, and *Haemophilus influenzae*.[5] By contrast, the central pathophysiology of CRS remains elusive to date. A variety of possible etiologic mechanisms have been proposed, including microbes (viruses, bacteria, fungi), allergy, osteitis, biofilm, staphylococcal superantigen, and derangements in innate and adaptive immunity. Although the exact role of bacteria in the disease process remains to be fully elucidated, it is likely that bacterial infection plays an important role in CRS, as either a causative or an exacerbating factor.[6]

### Differences in CRS and ARS Microbiology

The microbiology of CRS varies greatly from that of ARS. Nadel and colleagues[7] evaluated 507 endoscopically guided cultures in 265 patients. The predominant organisms identified included *Staphylococcus aureus* (31.3%), coagulase-negative *Staphylococcus* (SCN) (44.2%), and gram-negative rods (34.3%). A multitude of gram-negative organisms were cultured, with the most common being *Pseudomonas aeruginosa*, *Stenotrophomonas maltophilia*, *Escherichia coli*, and *Serratia marcescens*. Kingdom and Swain[8] analyzed 182 total cultures with 257 isolates in 101 patients at the time of sinus surgery. The microbiological yield was similar; the most common isolates were SCN (45%), gram-negative rods (25%), and *S aureus* (24%). Comparative analysis between primary and revision sinus surgery cases demonstrated no differences in bacterial yield or types. Bhattacharyya and Gopal[9] have demonstrated that whereas approximately half of the bacteria cultured in CRS are found in isolation, the rest exhibit polymicrobial growth, with 2 or more bacterial species.

## STAPHYLOCOCCUS AUREUS

*S aureus* is a ubiquitous microorganism, occupying the nasal vestibule of nearly one-third of the human population at any given time. *S aureus* has emerged as an important pathogen in community-acquired and hospital-acquired infections, resulting in sepsis, bacteremia, endocarditis, and soft-tissue infections. *S aureus* is commonly assayed in cultures performed for CRS.[7,8,10,11] Nadel and colleagues[7] and Kingdom and Swain[8] reported its presence in 23.1% and 25% of all cultures, respectively. Though the exact role in pathogenesis is a matter of debate, the presence of S aureus infection at the time of sinus surgery has been demonstrated to be a strong predictor of postoperative S aureus infection and impaired mucosal healing.

### Biofilms and Other Novel Mechanisms of Pathogenicity

A variety of novel mechanisms of pathogenicity have also been implicated, including biofilm formation, intracellular residency, and toxin-mediated disease.[12] Foreman and colleagues[13] characterized bacterial biofilm by fluorescence in situ hybridization in 50 CRS patients. Biofilms were detected in 36 of 50 patients, with S aureus being the most common biofilm forming organism. The capacity to form biofilms may confer the ability to create a recalcitrant infectious milieu unresponsive to conventional antimicrobial therapies. Further, enterotoxins derived from S aureus have been implicated in the pathophysiology of nasal polyps as disease-modifying factors.[14]

### Methicillin-Resistant S aureus in ARS and CRS

An increase in the recovery of methicillin-resistant S aureus (MRSA) has recently been noted in acute and CRS and anterior nares of normal individuals. Brook and colleagues[15] compared MRSA rates in chronic maxillary sinusitis between two time periods. S aureus was found in 15 (15%) of the patients between 2001 and 2003, 4 (27%) of which were MRSA. S aureus was cultured in 23 (20%) of the patients between 2004 and 2006, with 14 (61%) being MRSA. Indeed, MRSA represents a treatment challenge in the setting of CRS, given the paucity of optimal treatment options. Oral antibiotics that may be effective include doxycycline, trimethoprim/sulfamethoxazole, and clindamycin. Topical mupirocin irrigations may also serve as an important adjunct in the postoperative CRS patient.[16] This scenario suggests that a high index of suspicion must be maintained for the presence of MRSA sinusitis; endoscopically guided cultures are imperative in guiding targeted oral and/or topical antimicrobial therapy.

## COAGULASE-NEGATIVE STAPHYLOCOCCUS

The exact role of SCN in CRS remains to be elucidated, as its reported incidence varies widely.[8] It has been posited to be a contaminant, supported by previous work that found SCN in the middle meatus of 56% of healthy patients and in only 20% of patients with CRS.[17] Moreover, the microbe is ubiquitous on human skin, thus contamination may occur readily in the absence of proper sterile precautions during culture technique. However, different strains of SCN may have differing abilities to cause disease.

Recent studies evaluating SCN in indwelling devices have shown that bacterial pathogenicity is dependent on genes associated with biofilm formation, which are only found in certain strains.[18] The presence of SCN may not indicate infection, as a specific strain may be necessary for such an infection to develop. Nonetheless, endoscopically acquired cultures have consistently identified SCN in multiple studies in CRS. Bolger[10] found SCN in 17%, Hsu and colleagues[11] found SCN in 42%, and Nadel and colleagues[7] found SCN in 35% of cultures.[10,11]

One possible method to ascertain the significance of SCN culture is based on the quantitative growth on culture, along with presence of leukocytosis on the Gram stain result. Scant or light growth, especially with paucity of gram-positive rods or white blood cells (WBCs) on Gram stain, likely represents contamination. By contrast, moderate to heavy growth, with a large number of WBCs on Gram stain, should alert the clinician of the possibility of a true infection.

## PSEUDOMONAS AERUGINOSA

Gram-negative rods are often identified in CRS cultures, more commonly in patients who have undergone endoscopic sinus surgery.[7,10,11] However, their role in patients with CRS without previous surgery should also not be underestimated. Kingdom and Swain[8] found gram-negative rods in 31% of cultures in a group of patients at the time of primary sinus surgery. Nadel and colleagues[7] found gram-negative rods in 9.5% of cultures taken from patients without previous sinus surgery. P aeruginosa has long been recognized as an important pathogen in the upper and lower airway in patients with cystic fibrosis. It also represents a common and problematic organism in CRS. Rates of assay in CRS cultures have been reported as between 9% and 16%.[7,8] Nadel and colleagues[7] noted that that P aeruginosa was most commonly cultured in patients with previous FESS and irrigation usage. P aeruginosa also has the capability of biofilm formation, which may in part contribute to its refractory nature in CRS patients. Furthermore, the presence of P aeruginosa biofilm has been associated with poor evolution after FESS.[19] Fluoroquinolones are the only orally administered antibiotic group with efficacy against

*P aeruginosa*. Quinolone resistance has become more problematic, with limited alternative proven oral antimicrobial therapies for *Pseudomonas* rhinosinusitis.

## STENOTROPHOMONAS MALTOPHILIA

*S maltophilia* is a multidrug-resistant gram-negative bacillus most often encountered as a nosocomial pathogen in immunocompromised and intensive care unit patients. Infection with *S maltophilia* most frequently involves the respiratory tract, bloodstream, wounds, and genitourinary tract. *S maltophilia* has also been cultured from the paranasal sinuses, often in the setting of prior antimicrobial treatment and sinus surgery. The exact implication of *S maltophilia* cultures in the paranasal sinuses is unclear. Whether this represents a true infection by an atypical microorganism or colonization that surfaces after eradication of other microbes by antimicrobial therapy deserves additional research. Despite its multidrug-resistant nature, the use of trimethoprim/sulfamethoxazole and fluoroquinolone monotherapy has shown improvement of symptoms and endoscopic findings in CRS patients.[20]

## TRENDS IN BACTERIAL RESISTANCE

Antibiotic therapy is often used as an essential component of the comprehensive management strategy in the initial treatment of CRS and recurrent acute exacerbations of CRS. However, increased antibiotic exposure results in the potential for antibiotic resistance, which is especially problematic in patients with a chronic disease process, not infrequently requiring long-term medical therapy. As such, it is important to understand trends in antibiotic resistance in CRS, as this may have important clinical consequences in the ability to manage CRS.

Bhattacharyya and Kepnes[21] retrospectively reviewed a microbiological database to extract all endoscopically obtained cultures in adult patients with CRS from 2001 to 2005. A total of 701 bacterial isolates were reported. *S aureus* was the most commonly isolated organism (19%). Overall, antibiotic resistance significantly increased for erythromycin throughout the study, with a maximum resistance rate of 69.7%. Resistance remained unchanged for methicillin, clindamycin, levofloxacin, and sulfamethoxazole. Overall, 19% of *S aureus* species expressed methicillin resistance. MRSA species exhibited statistically significantly higher rates of resistance to other antibiotics tested compared with non-MRSA bacteria. The increasing resistance to erythromycin may have been due to

the trend to use macrolide antibiotics for their immunomodulatory, as well as antimicrobial, effect. This possibility does not necessarily indicate a resistance to macrolides as a class, but indicates poor effectiveness of erythromycin itself. While the rate of methicillin resistance among all bacteria evaluated (not only *S aureus*) remained stable, it still averaged greater than 30%, showing declining efficacy of first-generation cephalosporins.

These results are further corroborated in the previous work by Kingdom and Swain,[8] who noted high rates of quinolone resistance for SCN (21% of patients) and *S aureus* (21% of patients). Also, the high rate of resistance to methicillin was further exemplified among *S aureus* isolates in 21% of patients. Lastly, *P aeruginosa* isolates showed a 27% resistance rate to quinolones and 36% resistance rate to aminoglycosides.

Guss and colleagues[22] retrospectively reviewed all bacterial sinus cultures from a tertiary care rhinology practice that yielded *P aeruginosa* over a 5-year period. A total of 689 culture results from 324 patients were examined. Overall, 13% of all *P aeruginosa* cultured were resistant to levofloxacin, with 5% intermediately sensitive. Moreover, 5% were resistant to ciprofloxacin while 7% were intermediately sensitive. The resistance rates remained stable throughout the 5-year study period. The use of endoscopically derived cultures was crucial in ascertaining this high rate of fluoroquinolone resistance, supporting the use of culture-specific therapy.

## SUMMARY

This snapshot of bacteriologic data highlights the inherent difficulties in managing the infectious aspects of CRS. Although SCN, *S aureus*, and *P aeruginosa* predominate in microbiological studies, a multitude of gram-negative rods and other atypical organisms may also be cultures in refractory CRS, especially in the setting of previous sinus surgery. Selective pressures posed by antimicrobial therapy and the emergence of antibiotic resistance further add to the complexity of the management strategy. Thus, indiscriminate use of broad-spectrum antibiotic therapy should be discouraged. Targeted use of antibiotic therapy, specifically for infectious exacerbations of CRS based on endoscopically guided cultures, is preferable. A careful, judicious strategy will optimize the care of the aesthetic and reconstructive surgery patients when medical and surgical management of CRS is required concurrently with rhinoplasty or in a staged manner.

# REFERENCES

1. National Center for Health Statistics. National ambulatory medical care survey 1990-1995. Hyattsville (MD): US Public Health Service; 1997. Series 13 [CD-ROM].

2. Bhattacharyya N. Ambulatory sinus and nasal surgery in the United States: demographics and perioperative outcomes. Laryngoscope 2010;120: 635–8.

3. Fakhri S, Citardi MJ. Considerations against concurrent functional endoscopic sinus surgery and rhinoplasty. Facial Plast Surg Clin North Am 2004;12: 431–4.

4. McGraw-Wall B, MacGregor AR. Concurrent functional endoscopic sinus surgery and rhinoplasty: pros. Facial Plast Surg Clin North Am 2004;12: 425–9.

5. Brook I. Microbiology of sinusitis. Proc Am Thorac Soc 2011;8:90–100.

6. Biel MA, Brown CA, Levinson RM, et al. Evaluation of the microbiology of chronic maxillary sinusitis. Ann Otol Rhinol Laryngol 1998;107:942–5.

7. Nadel DM, Lanza DC, Kennedy DW. Endoscopically guided cultures in chronic sinusitis. Am J Rhinol 1998;12:233–41.

8. Kingdom TT, Swain RE. The microbiology and antimicrobial resistance patterns in chronic rhinosinusitis. Am J Otolaryngol 2004;25:323–8.

9. Bhattacharyya N, Gopal HV. Microbiology of the ethmoid sinus following endoscopic sinus surgery. Ear Nose Throat J 2002;81:558–61.

10. Bolger WE. Gram negative sinusitis: an emerging clinical entity? Am J Rhinol 1994;8:279–84.

11. Hsu J, Lanza DC, Kennedy DW. Antimicrobial resistance in bacterial chronic sinusitis. Am J Rhinol 1998;12:243–7.

12. Lowy FD. Staphylococcal aureus infections. N Engl J Med 1998;339:520–32.

13. Foreman A, Psaltis AJ, Tan LW, et al. Characterization of bacterial and fungal biofilms in chronic rhinosinusitis. Am J Rhinol Allergy 2009;23:556–61.

14. Bachert C, Zhang N, Patou J, et al. Role of staphylococcal superantigens in upper airway disease. Curr Opin Allergy Clin Immunol 2008;8:34–8.

15. Brook I, Foote PA, Hausfeld JN. Increase in the frequency of recovery of methicillin-resistant *Staphylococcus aureus* in acute and chronic maxillary sinusitis. J Med Microbiol 2008;57:1015–7.

16. Solares CA, Batra PS, Hall GS, et al. Treatment of chronic rhinosinusitis exacerbations due to methicillin-resistant *Staphylococcus aureus* with mupirocin irrigation. Am J Otolaryngol 2006;27:161–5.

17. Araujo E, Palombini BC, Cantarelli V, et al. Microbiology of middle meatus in chronic rhinosinusitis. Am J Rhinol 2003;17:9–15.

18. Larson DA, Han JK. Microbiology of sinusitis: does allergy or endoscopic sinus surgery affect the microbiologic flora? Curr Opin Otolaryngol Head Neck Surg 2011;19(3):199–203.

19. Bendouah Z, Barbeau J, Hamad WA, et al. Biofilm formation by *Staphylococcus aureus* and *Pseudomonas aeruginosa* is associated with an unfavorable evolution after surgery for chronic sinusitis and nasal polyposis. Otolaryngol Head Neck Surg 2006;134: 991–6.

20. Grindler D, Thomas C, Hall GS, et al. The role of *Stenotrophomonas maltophilia* in refractory chronic rhinosinusitis. Am J Rhinol Allergy 2010; 24:200–4.

21. Bhattacharyya N, Kepnes LJ. Assessment of trends in antimicrobial resistance in chronic rhinosinusitis. Ann Otol Rhinol Laryngol 2008;117: 448–52.

22. Guss J, Abuzeid WM, Doghramji L, et al. Fluoroquinolone-resistant *Pseudomonas aeruginosa* in chronic rhinosinusitis. ORL J Otorhinolaryngol Relat Spec 2009;71:263–7.

# Smell and Taste Disorders

Terah J. Allis, MD, Donald A. Leopold, MD*

## KEYWORDS

- Smell disorders • Taste disorders • Olfactory disorders

---

**Key Points**

- Olfactory testing is crucial for accurately diagnosing chemosensory problems and before nasal surgery as a medical-legal safeguard for a medical practice. There are several easy-to-use smell and taste tests.
- Olfaction is a complex process involving both orthonasal and retronasal pathways for olfactory stimulation.
- The astute surgeon may identify nasal and systemic disease factors that may play a role in postoperative olfactory loss.
- The presence of functioning senses of taste and smell is a major boost to quality of life and safety.

---

The chemosenses of smell and taste contribute to quality of life and environmental appreciation. Not only do these senses guard against toxic and dangerous stimuli, but the ability to smell and taste contributes to the finer qualities of life, including participating in wine tasting, detecting a fresh-brewed steaming cup of coffee, or baking Christmas cookies. Nasal surgery can alter a patient's olfaction[1] and some patients have unrecognized olfactory loss before surgery. A recent study from Turkey found that practitioners who were educated about olfactory loss were more likely to rate smell loss as important and be more confident in managing smell loss.[2] We advocate that a basic smell test and record of a patient's olfaction before surgery is key to avoiding both patient injury and legal misfortune. A working knowledge and awareness of the many factors that contribute to a patient's sense of smell (and taste) is fundamental.

Surgeons must pay attention to surgical risk factors, surgical techniques, and existing preoperative disease because these can lead to olfactory disturbances and permanent smell loss after surgery.

## ANATOMY
### Olfaction

The organs of olfaction are unique within the human body because they contain neuroepithelium that regenerates. However, these delicate nerve fibers may also be damaged and undergo permanent loss. Grossly, the nasal passages contain the structures of olfaction, which include the upper nasal septum, and middle and superior turbinates. These structures facilitate airflow and contain the primary olfactory neurons. Olfactory molecules dissolve in mucous overlying these neurons and then interact with the neurons,

---

Funding and disclosures: No funding support was obtained. Dr Allis has no financial disclosures or conflicts of interest. Dr Leopold is a consultant for: Neilmed Corp; Entellus Medical, Inc; Optinose US, Inc.
Department of Otolaryngology–Head and Neck Surgery, University of Nebraska Medical Center, 981225 Nebraska Medical Center, Omaha, NE 68198-1225, USA
* Corresponding author.
E-mail address: dleopold@unmc.edu

Facial Plast Surg Clin N Am 20 (2012) 93–111
doi:10.1016/j.fsc.2011.10.011
1064-7406/12/$ – see front matter © 2012 Elsevier Inc. All rights reserved.

producing an action potential. The olfactory bulb, which is positioned at the anterior cranial fossa, serves as the initial transfer station in the olfactory pathway (**Fig. 1**). The primary olfactory neurons synapse with secondary neurons, which constitutes aggregates referred to as glomeruli.[3] The olfactory cleft lies in a protected location approximately 7 cm from the nasal sill (**Fig. 2**).[4] Olfactory bulb comes from the Latin words *olfactus*, which means sense of smell, and *bulbus*, which means swollen root. This region is where the olfactory nerves (cranial nerve I) terminate and the olfactory tracts arise.[5]

Cranial nerve I mediates the olfactory response with additional input from cranial nerves V, IX, and X. The trigeminal nerve relays pungent or irritating odors such as carbon dioxide, which is known to be a pure trigeminal stimulant. Cranial nerves IX and X assist in retronasal olfaction, which is further discussed in this article. The human olfactory epithelium covers an area of roughly 1 $cm^2$ on each side.[6] Humans have approximately 6 million olfactory neurons.[7]

### Vomeronasal Organ

In more than 80% of adults, there is a pit or cleft located in the anteroinferior nasal septum. This pit

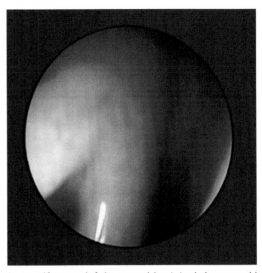

**Fig. 2.** Olfactory cleft (D. Leopold, original photograph).

contains neuroepithelium-like tissue that has no neural connection to the brain. Explanations for its existence include that is a vestigial olfactory organ (which functions in many other animals), or that it has a neuroendocrine function.[8,9] The data to date suggest that it has no functional significance.[10]

### Microhistology

The olfactory epithelium is primarily composed of pseudostratified columnar-type epithelium, is situated with a vascular lamina propria, and lacks a submucosa (**Fig. 3**). The cells that facilitate olfaction are divided into 4 main cell types: ciliated olfactory receptors, microvillar cells, sustentacular cells, and basal cells.[11–14] In the olfactory mucosa, the axons from the bipolar olfactory neurons coalesce into bundles to form cranial nerve I (**Fig. 4**). This nerve traverses upward through the cribriform plate and skull base to the olfactory bulb. A complex olfactory map brings signals to higher processing centers, which is thought to be partly responsible for olfactory coding.[15,16]

### Clinical Olfaction

#### Definitions

Loss of the sense of smell is subdivided into categories dependent on the degree of loss, dysfunction, or altered perception. It is important to correctly identify and document the type of loss or dysfunction because each has distinct prognosis and treatments.

- Normosmia is used to describe the perception of an intact sense of smell

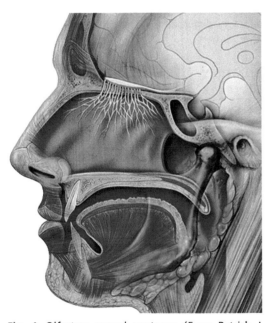

**Fig. 1.** Olfactory neural anatomy. (*From* Patrick J. Lynch C. Carl Jaffe. Cardiologist, Yale University Center for Advanced Instructional Media. Medical illustrations by Patrick Lynch, generated for multimedia teaching projects by the Yale University School of Medicine, Center for Advanced Instructional Media, 1987–2000; with permission.)

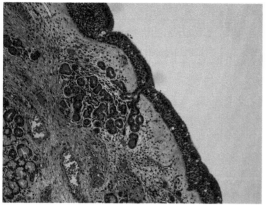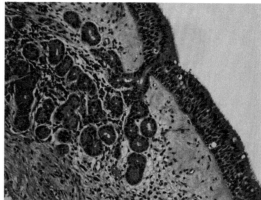

Fig. 3. Microhistology of olfactory epithelium. (*Courtesy of* Dr E. Linde, Department of Pathology, UNMC.)

- Hyposmia describes a decreased ability to perceive smell
- Anosmia describes the absence of useful smelling ability
- Parosmia is the distorted perception of odor following a stimulus
- Phantosmia is perception of odor in the absence of an odorant stimulus.

## Taste

### Definitions

Most patient-described losses or disturbances of taste are olfactory losses. True solitary taste loss is less common.

- Hypogeusia is diminished sense of taste
- Ageusia is absence of taste
- Dysgeusia is altered or distorted taste sensation.

### Taste (Gustatory) Anatomy

The oral cavity contains taste receptors (taste buds within papilla) largely on the tongue but also on the palate, pharynx, and epiglottis. Grossly, the tongue is composed of multiple taste papillae geographically distributed. Fungiform, circumvallate, and foliate papillae contain taste buds that facilitate gustatory sensation (**Fig. 5**). The filiform papillas do not contribute to taste but

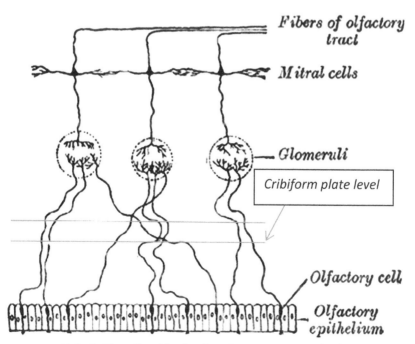

Fig. 4. Olfactory neurons. (*Adapted from* Standring S, editor. Gray's anatomy. 40th edition. Philadelphia: Churchill Livingstone; 2008; with permission.)

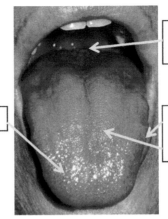

Circumvallate papillae
(more posteriorly)

Fungiform papillae

Foliate papillae (superior arrow)

Filiform papillae (inferior arrow)

**Fig. 5.** Tongue and taste bud anatomy (Courtesy of T. Allis MD, Omaha, NE.).

are readily distributed in the tongue.[17] The chorda tympani (cranial nerve VII) mediates taste from the anterior two-thirds of the tongue. The glossopharyngeal nerve (cranial nerve IX) mediates the posterior one-third of the tongue and circumvallate papilla. The vagus facilitates sensation from the posterior pharynx and laryngeal epiglottis. Taste neurons also regenerate, and are replaced approximately every 10 days.

## PHYSIOLOGY OF SMELL

Nasal airflow plays an integral part of smell detection. Although olfactory particles can contact the olfactory cleft by diffusion, airflow is generally a prerequisite of olfaction. As airflow distributes itself in the nasal cavity, about 15% flows to the olfactory cleft (**Fig. 6**). Smell is typically thought of as being mediated through nasal inhalation with orthonasal flow. Another contributor to

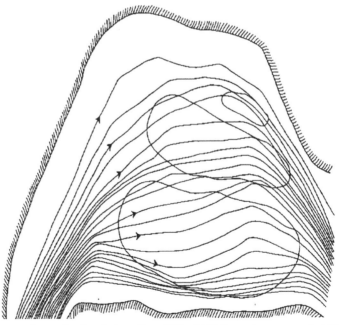

**Fig. 6.** Streamline patterns for resting inspiratory flow (250 mL/s/s) through an expanded (20× normal size) scale model of a healthy human adult male nasal cavity (sagittal view). Lines show the paths taken by small dust particles entering at the external nares. (*From* Scherer PW, Scherer PW, Hahn II, et al. The biophysics of nasal airflow. Otolaryngol Clin North Am 1989;22:265; with permission.)

olfaction and food flavor perception is retronasal olfaction, which occurs during ingestion of substances with airflow of odorant molecules generated by exhalation, or mouth and pharynx contraction. This phenomenon is important clinically because a group of patients display adequate retronasal olfactory function with modest or no orthonasal function remaining, and yet these patients recognize smell. The differences between orthonasal and retronasal perception of odor are at least partly caused by absorption of odors to the olfactory epithelium, which seems to differ in relation to the direction of the airflow across the olfactory epithelium. This concept favors a duality of smell.[18–21]

Inherently, key to this process is that odorant molecules must dissolve in or pass through the mucous overlying the olfactory epithelium to be detected. Once the odorants bind to the receptor neurons, a complex enzyme-mediated pathway ensues (**Fig. 7**).[22] This chemical and electrical pathway transmits neuronal information to higher centers involving both the frontal lobes and temporal lobes. These pathways are complex and interweaving, allowing humans to associate memories with a particular smell and event.[23–25] For example, the smell of a fir tree makes many people recall Christmas time.

## PHYSIOLOGY OF TASTE

Traditionally, taste is subdivided into 5 major gustatory classifications: salty, sweet, bitter, sour, and umami. In the taste buds, the chemical molecules are transformed into electrical signals that travel to the nucleus solitarius (medulla), to the ventricular posterior medial nucleus in the thalamus and to the parietal lobe, and give the perception of gustation.

Another integral component of gustation is the pleasure related to the oral sensation and tastes of the food ingested. Genetics play a role in what is interpreted as pleasurable, and obesity has been linked with the feel of foods.[26] A group of receptors, T1R1-3s, have been found to detect sweet tastes. Conversely, the taste of certain foods protect from toxins and other harmful substances, and an even larger collection of T2R receptors facilitates bitter taste sensation.[27] A sensation dependent on the lipid content of the food, described as fatty taste, may increase the pleasantness derived from tasting food.[28–30] This sensation has been studied in rats and miceand has been linked to circumvallate papillae function.[30]

## DIAGNOSIS AND WORKUP OF OLFACTORY COMPLAINTS
### Clinical History of Olfactory or Taste Loss

A discussion with the patient while obtaining a history is useful for identifying the onset, symptoms, and duration of smell and taste changes. The patient may not disclose an olfactory disturbance unless directly asked. Associated clinical clues such as preceding trauma or viral infection are helpful in determining the cause of the perceived loss. According to rough projections, at least 1% of patients have an unrecognized loss.[31] One study found that up to 16% of the general population has an olfactory disturbance.[32] Patients may also complain of taste disturbance instead of an olfactory loss, which should increase the surgeon's suspicion of a probable smell disturbance because the 2 senses are intimately linked.

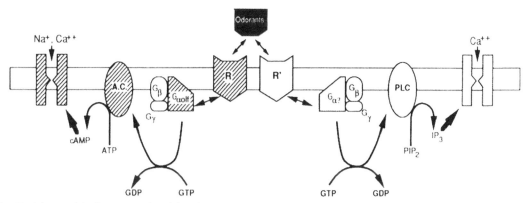

**Fig. 7.** Odorant binding. AC, adenylyl cyclase; ATP, adenosine triphosphate; CaBP, calmodulin-binding protein; cAMP, cyclic adenosine monophosphate; CNG channel, cyclic nucleotide–gated channel; ORK, olfactory receptor kinase; PDE, phosphodiesterase; PKA, protein kinase A; RGS, regulator of G proteins (but here acts on the AC). Arrows indicate stimulatory and inhibitory (feedback) pathways. (*From* Firestein S. How the olfactory system makes sense of scents. Nature 2001;413:211. Reprinted by permission from Macmillan Publishers Ltd.)

A brief discussion of medications for association with dysgeusia is also warranted.

### Physical Examination for Olfaction

The facial plastic surgeon will assess the patient's nose for aesthetics and functional deformities, dimensions, and collapsibility of skin, cartilage, and nasal valve. A brief examination of the nasal cavity on anterior rhinoscopy may reveal gross disease such as septal perforation, polyps, systemic disease, and epistaxis, tumors, or allergic edematous nasal mucosa. Documentation of the physical examination is vital before surgery. Neurologic status and cranial nerve function should be assessed. If the surgeon performs nasal endoscopy, a view of the olfactory cleft and assessment of blockage may predict olfactory dysfunction.[4] Tumors or polyps may also be ruled out on highly sensitive nasal endoscopy. A comprehensive description of appropriate workup is given in **Fig. 8**.

## CHEMOSENSORY TESTING
### Olfactory Testing

Two classes of testing are available: electrophysical and psychophysical tests; however, psychophysical tests are more useful in the interoffice setting, more widely used, simple, and easy for the plastic rhinoplasty surgeon to use.[33] Electrophysical tests are generally reserved for research studies. Testing olfaction documents not only the extent of the olfactory loss but also allows for comparisons during clinical follow-up and assessment for improvement over time (duration of deficit). Olfactory testing generally measures either threshold of smell or identification of various smells.[4] A wide variety of tests are available in the olfactory work-up. Surgeons working on or around the nose should be familiar with the benefits and disadvantages of these tests (**Table 1**).

### Alcohol pad test

Perhaps the simplest tests include the use of an isopropyl alcohol wipe pad to detect degrees of hyposmia or anosmia. The patient with eyes closed has an alcohol pad slowly brought from a distance to close to the nose. The patient states when the odor is first perceived, and this distance from the examiner and alcohol pad correlates with the degree of olfactory loss (see **Table 1**).[34] The test has been able to differentiate hyposmic and anosmic patients and can be modified for unilateral testing.

### Odorant tests

Threshold tests with different odorants, most commonly pyridine and n-butyl alcohol (1-butanol),

and phenylethyl alcohol rose smell (less trigeminal stimulation than the others), test the patient's detection threshold at different concentrations ranging from the least concentrated to the most concentrated odorant. The patient may also be presented with either a bottle containing the odorant or a placebo and be asked to choose the one with the odorant.[35,36] Drawbacks to this test are low test-retest reliability, the time required for testing, and the need for a tester.[37,38]

Smell identification tests are used worldwide and are available with culture-specific data. Microencapsulated odorants make these tests easy for self-administration (**Fig. 9**). The patient is presented with suprathreshold levels of odorants and asked to correctly identify the various odorants. Normative age-related and sex-related data via percentages are accessible. Countries such as Brazil and Australia have developed their own normative data.[39–41]

In other parts of the world, olfactory testing is also being performed, sometimes with one of the tests noted previously and sometimes with locally designed tests.[42] In Japan, the standard test is the T&T olfactometer, which is a rack containing 8 concentrations of 5 different odorants. From this test, both detection and recognition thresholds can be determined, and they are charted on a graph similar to an audiogram.[42]

In Germany, an odorant threshold and identification forced-choice test that uses odorant-impregnated felt-tip pens has been developed. It can be reused and has short test administration times (**Fig. 10**).[43]

### Computed tomography scans

If the history, physical examination, or olfactory tests suggest polypoid or obstructive disease or malignant potential, then sinonasal imaging is completed. Computed tomography (CT) scans of the paranasal region, principally in the coronal plane, are beneficial in assessing any anatomic abnormalities, tumors, malignancy, or obstructive disorder. Bony definition is particularly well defined on CT scan.[4] Magnetic resonance imaging (MRI) gives an inadequate portrayal of bony detail, but may visualize the olfactory sulci and brain structure.[44–46]

## CLINICAL EVALUATION OF TASTE
### History

Patients presenting with a complaint of taste disturbance should be asked about any associated disorder of smell; any preexisting medical conditions and their treatment, such as ear infection, ear surgery, Bell palsy, significant head injury,

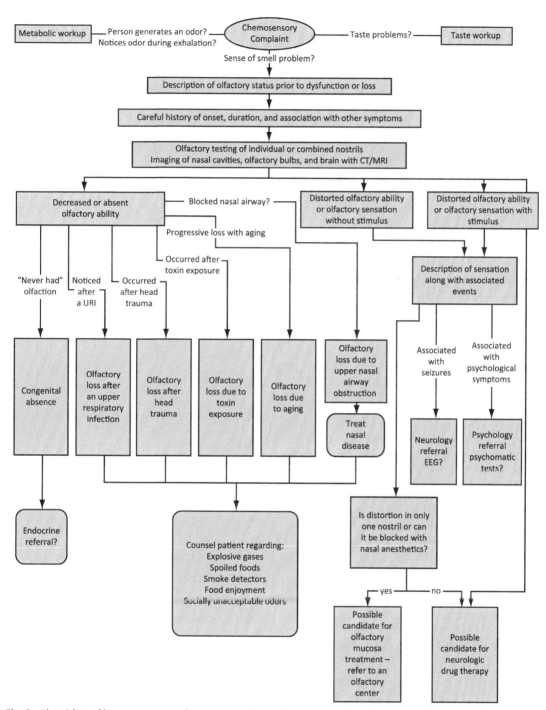

**Fig. 8.** Algorithm of how to manage the patient with an olfactory disorder. CT, computed tomography; EEG, electroencephalography; MRI, magnetic resonance imaging; URI, upper respiratory tract infection. (*From* Holbrook E, Leopold DA. Physiology of olfaction. In: Flint PW, Haughey BH, Lund VJ, et al, editors. Cummings otolaryngology head and neck surgery, 5th edition. Philadelphia: Mosby; 2010. chapter 41, Figure 41-14; with permission.)

recent upper respiratory tract illness, and various dental procedures or prostheses.[47] A detailed medication history also should be obtained.

In addition to a physical examination and testing of taste and smell, special attention should be paid to the oral cavity for evidence of infection, inflammation, degeneration, and masses, as well as atrophy and dryness of tongue, gums, dentition, and surrounding mucous membranes. Specific investigations are ordered to identify suspected

**Table 1**
**Various types of olfactory testing**

| Name | Type | Advantages | Disadvantages |
|------|------|-----------|---------------|
| Alcohol pad | Threshold | Quick, simple, inexpensive, can test unilateral function | Less rigorous |
| Threshold tests (pyridine) | Threshold | Simple | Low test-retest reliability, time intensive |
| Smell identification tests | Identification, suprathreshold | Compares normative data, fun, portable, test for malingering | Requires grading |
| Sniffin' sticks | Threshold and identification | Reusable, rapid administration | Availability, expensive |
| T & T olfactometer | Threshold | Standardized in Japan, graph data | More labor intensive |

causative considerations suggested by the clinical features. If no local cause is suggested, patients with taste abnormalities, particularly unilateral, should undergo audiologic evaluation and imaging studies to include the middle ear.

The sense of taste can be tested with readily available stimuli, such as aqueous solutions of sugar, sodium chloride, acetic acid, and quinine, or with electrical stimulation of the tongue (electrogustometry). A cotton applicator is used to rub the aqueous solution gently onto the lateral quadrant of the protruded tongue. The patient should not withdraw the protruded tongue, close the mouth, or talk, but should identify the perceived taste by pointing to cards printed with the words sweet, salt, sour, and bitter. The mouth is then rinsed with water between tests. Electrogustometry is the evaluation of taste by applying graded electrical currents to the tongue to produce a sensation described as sour or metallic. In normal subjects, the 2 sides of the tongue have similar thresholds for electrical stimulation, rarely differing by more than 25%. The technique has the advantages of simplicity, speed, and ease of quantification, and is capable of providing a reliable objective recording of the gustatory detection threshold.[47]

## Common Causes of Olfactory Loss

Disorders of olfaction are common worldwide and may involve as many as 2 to 4 million people in the United States.[31] As previously defined, wide variations occur in perceptions of smell, and testing is available to assist in delineation of the degree of loss. Olfactory disturbances can be better separated into those with a conductive component (anatomic blockage of the olfactory cleft or surrounding structures) and a sensorineural component (a nerve loss or damage to receptor or higher cortical processing). This distinction

is important for distinguishing those who have chance of improvement and treatment. Generally, conductive losses are treatable.

## Conductive Losses (Nasal Obstructions)

### Nasal inflammatory disease
Nasal inflammatory disease encompasses a variety of nasal disorders from chronic rhinosinusitis to polyps or allergic edema. This group of disorders is thought to primarily alter nasal airflow to the olfactory cleft; however, there is evidence that a sensorineural component and changes in the neural olfactory epithelium on histologic examination can occur (**Fig. 11**).[48,49]

## NEURAL LOSSES
### After Upper Respiratory Infection

Many patients report temporary decreased smell during upper respiratory infection (URI), which is largely mediated by acute nasal edema and decrease of airflow during a viral infection. The nasal membrane edema commonly abates within a few days and smell returns to baseline. However, in a subset of patients, there is permanent olfactory loss following URI and the prognosis is principally poor, with only one-third recovering.[50] In these patients a sensorineural insult occurs to the primary olfactory neurons.[51] Olfactory cleft biopsies usually show a complete loss of olfactory receptors or fewer numbers.[52–54] The olfactory bulb shows atrophy over time.[52] Olfactory bulb scans in these patients reveals a decrease in size that correlates with severity of loss as well as duration of the hyposmia.[52] The individuals affected by this tend to be otherwise healthy individuals in the fourth, fifth, or sixth decade of life, and they are overwhelmingly women (70%–80%).[50,55–57] The reason for this female preponderance is unclear

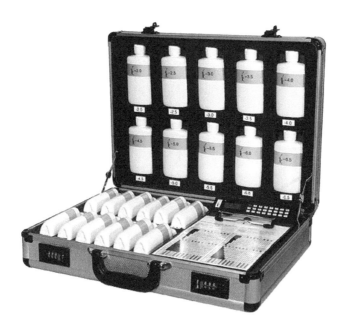

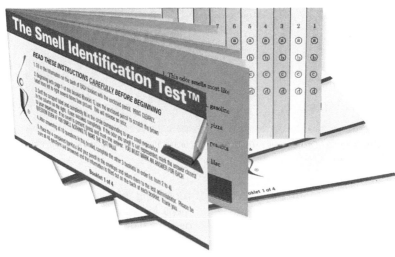

**Fig. 9.** Smell identification test (*Courtesy of* Sensonics, Inc., Haddon Heights, NJ. © 2011 Sensonics, Inc; with permission.)

but may relate to women tending to have more URIs.[58]

Although the mechanism of permanent olfactory dysfunction after URI remains indeterminate, recent research alludes to more than apoptosis of olfactory neurons with peripheral anatomic changes such as scarring or central processing dysfunction.[59] Agents such as minocycline (thought to inhibit apoptosis) have been administered to patients with anosmia or hyposmia without associated benefit.[59]

The prognosis for recovery from this olfactory loss is generally poor and there is no effective treatment. Hendriks[50] combined several reported studies of patients with olfactory dysfunction and found that approximately one-third of the patients recovered their olfactory ability.

### Head Trauma and Loss of Smell

About 5% to 10% of patients with head trauma suffer from smell loss, often from occipital or frontal blows.[60–63] The location of cranial trauma is related to the degree of olfactory loss. Frontal blows more commonly result in loss of olfactory function, whereas occipital trauma is more likely to cause total anosmia.[50,64] The mechanism is thought to be related to shearing at the level

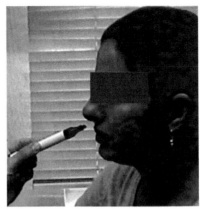

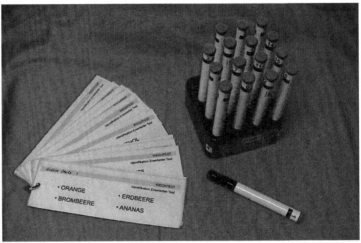

**Fig. 10.** Sniffin' sticks. (Photo *Courtesy of* Dr Hummel, Sniffin' Sticks, Burghart Modizintechnik, Erlangen, Germany.)

of the cribriform plate, injury to the olfactory bulb, or supraorbital and frontal brain contusions that result in axonal injury.[65]

### Aging and Loss of Smell

Olfactory loss is a known entity with aging; however, the astute clinician is also aware that neurocognitive diseases in the elderly, such as Alzheimer and Parkinson, may also manifest with olfactory dysfunction. The sense of smell has been studied and defined with age-related norms and known decreases, especially in individuals more than 65 years of age.[66] This decline in function is similar to age-related visual acuity changes.[67] As expected, with advanced age there is olfactory bulb volume loss.[68]

### Congenital Loss of Smell

Patients who suffer from anosmia caused by a congenital absence perform the poorest on smell tests.[56,69] Absence of receptors and

supporting cells is seen on histopathology specimens in this group. The cause is secondary to degeneration or failure of formation of the olfactory bulb and/or epithelium during development.[69] These patients often present around 8 years of

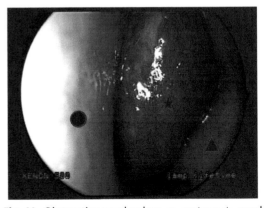

**Fig. 11.** Obstructive nasal polyps. ●, septum; ★, nasal polyp; ▲, inferior turbinate, which is pushed laterally by the polyp (Courtesy of D. Leopold, Omaha, NE.).

age with anosmia.[69] The most recognized congenital disorder is Kallman syndrome or hypogonadotropic hypogonadism.[70,71] Kallman syndrome is caused by a mutation in KAL1 (sporadic) or KAL2 (autosomal dominant) and results in at least partial loss of the olfactory bulbs and stalks, incomplete development of the hypothalamus,[72–74] or lack of olfactory epithelium.[69] A coronal CT or MRI scan often shows a flat skull base anteriorly with no dip into the nasal cavity (Katherine Johnson, Leight W, Wood JW, Leopold DA. Evaluation of Keros score in patients with congenital anosmia, Manuscript to be published, personal communication, May 2011).

## Toxins and Loss of Smell

Toxic exposure and subsequent olfactory dysfunction is best described as a sensorineural injury. There remains an extensive list of toxins composed of classes of metals, gases, and solvents that are known to be harmful to olfaction. Substances range from acetone and tobacco to cadmium and silicosis and cotton.[75] However, this subgroup of olfactory disorders only comprises between 1% and 5% of olfactory disorders.[76] The diagnosis is largely based on history and known environmental exposure to the toxin. The nasal mucosa has a high-blood-perfusion region that may contribute to the toxin's effects besides that of direct contact or inhalation. Overall, the effects are not well understood and there are no treatments available besides removal of the toxic exposure. Prevention and education are key.

## Neoplasm and Loss of Smell

Another group that may be both conductive deficit and sensorineural, based on location, are nasal, paranasal sinus, skull base tumors, and intracranial tumors. These tumors often block airflow and sense of smell unilaterally; however, intracranial meningiomas, gliomas, and other tumors may cause confined destruction of the central olfactory neurons.[4] The intranasal tumors most frequently encountered are inverting papillomas, adenomas, squamous cell carcinomas, and esthesioneuroblastomas.[77] About one-quarter of temporal lobe neoplasms have related olfactory disturbance.[78]

## Postsurgery Loss of Smell

### Nasal surgery

Surgery at or near to the structures of olfaction can result in alteration in smell. If surgeons do not test and document olfactory loss at baseline, they can miss a loss before surgery. Hyposmia or anosmia

after nasal surgery are typically caused by 4 mechanisms (**Table 2**)[79]:

1. Scar tissue
2. Granulation tissue
3. Persistent mucosal edema
4. Inflammation and olfactory neuroepithelial damage

Numerous studies have documented a small, but important, permanent loss in smell after surgery. Septoplasty, turbinectomy or reduction, rhinoplasty, functional sinus surgery, and laryngectomy are among the more common surgical procedures whereby olfaction can be worsened. The mechanisms for each type of surgery are described later. Olfactory loss has also been reported with general anesthesia.[79–81]

### Middle turbinate resection

Kimmelman[1] suggested that a resection of the lower half of the middle turbinate likely does not result in anosmia or hyposmia, although injury to the olfactory epithelium that covers the superior portions of the middle turbinate is possible. A study completed by Biedlingmaier and colleagues[82] reviewed patients with partial middle turbinate resections during routine sinus surgery. They found that only 1 patient out of 198 (0.9%) complained of anosmia, 1 patient experienced bleeding that required surgical control, and no patients had evidence of crusting.[82] This anosmia rate is similar to the 0.8% rate with preservation of the middle turbinate.[83]

### Septoplasty complications

Overall, olfactory dysfunction after surgery is rare after septoplasty,[84] although, in the acute postoperative period, a transient decrease in smell may be experienced because of mucosal edema and altered air flow. One study found that total anosmia following septoplasty in the long term was found in 0.3% to 2.9% and hyposmia 1%. However, olfactory disturbance may be present in up to 8% of patients before septoplasty, and both the surgeon and patient may be unaware without preoperative testing.[85] Rettinger and Kirshe[84] recommended preoperative smell test/threshold tests because of the possibility of scarring, adhesions, and changes of airflow directions. Another study by Pade and Hummel[86] suggested that, in patients undergoing septoplasty, only 10% experienced an improvement in olfaction after surgery. They noted that a small number of patients who had high preoperative functioning showed decreased postoperative olfaction. The investigators therefore recommended appropriate

**Table 2**
**Mechanisms of olfactory loss from sinonasal surgery**

| Origin of Injury from Nasal Surgery | Explanation |
|---|---|
| Mechanical injury | Direct trauma to olfactory epithelium:<br>1. From electrocautery<br>2. Lasers (direct or scatter)<br>3. Traction on the olfactory filia caused by cribriform plate kinesis (superior septoplasty, high osteotomies)<br>4. Abrasion<br>Scarring or mechanical occlusion in olfactory region<br>Atrophic rhinitis (higher risk after inferior turbinectomy), crusting, dryness |
| Airflow modification | Anatomic narrowing, widening, or scarring that alters flow to olfactory region |
| Vascular injury | Vascular compromise to olfactory neuroepithelium secondary to surgically created ischemia<br>Postoperative URI (herpes) |
| Neural injury | Vascular compromise to olfactory neuroepithelium secondary to surgically created ischemia, crush injury<br>Postoperative URI (herpes) |
| Postoperative medicines | Local anesthetics topical/injected<br>Topical zinc |
| Preoperative factors | Unrecognized preexisting anosmia/hyposmia |
| Psychological factors | Anxiety/stress |

*Adapted from* Wrobel BB, Leopold DA. Smell and taste disorders. Facial Plas Surg Clin N Am 2004;12(4):459–68; with permission.

preoperative counseling regarding potential smell loss.[86]

### Rhinoplasty complications

Smell dysfunction following rhinoplasty has been reported and studied. However, there remains a lack of randomized clinical trials assessing smell loss after rhinoplasty. Most of the reports are level III or IV cohort studies and case reports. One of the earliest studies, from the 1960s, is from Champion,[87] who analyzed 200 cases of rhinoplasty at between 6 and 18 months following surgery for subjective smell loss. In this study, no formal olfactory testing was completed. The investigator reported that 22 patients had temporary olfactory dysfunction and 1 patient had permanent anosmia. Another study analyzed 97 patients who underwent rhinoplasty or submucous resection and did perform olfactory testing with odorant bottles both before surgery and after surgery. Three patients had decreased olfactory function.[88] This suggests a low risk overall (~3%), but that it is nonetheless a risk that needs to be addressed with patients. In the study by Kimmelman,[1] patients undergoing a wide variety of sinus and nasal surgeries (94 patients total/ 15 rhinoplasty) were studied both before and after surgery with smell tests, and 34% had

decreased smell. **Table 2** illustrates the proposed pathophysiology/mechanism for surgical-related olfactory dysfunction. In summary, the literature clearly delineates a risk of hyposmia or anosmia with rhinoplasty, albeit a small risk.

### Skull base surgery and loss of smell

Complex anterior and middle fossa skull base surgery, and many cranial surgeries near the olfactory bulbs, may cause olfactory loss. In particular, surgical manipulation in close proximity to the olfactory tract has been connected with complete, permanent loss of olfactory capacity. Surgeons have developed endoscopic and less invasive techniques to spare the olfactory tissue.[89–91]

### Laryngectomy and loss of smell

After laryngectomy with loss of normal nasal airflow, most patients develop anosmia. Buccal or nasal airflow maneuvers can assist patients with gaining airflow and olfaction rehabilitation after surgery. In a study by Hilgers and colleagues,[92] by using the polite yawning technique (nasal airflow-inducing maneuver [NAIM]), up to 50% of patients were able to regain olfactory function. Evaluation with Sniffin' Sticks tests in patients after laryngectomy showed a clinically relevant increase of olfaction in 80% of patients in another study.[93] The teaching of the NAIM should be included in postlaryngectomy rehabilitation programs.

## Neurodegenerative Disorders and Loss of Smell

Much research has recently been devoted to the link between olfactory loss and neurodegenerative disorders such as Alzheimer disease and Parkinson disease. There exists an olfactory component to these disease processes and it often precedes the clinical diagnosis. It has been estimated that a decrease in olfactory function heralds the onset of motor symptoms in patients with Parkinson disease by roughly 4 years.[94,95] Identifying hyposmia has been characterized as a useful part of formulating the diagnosis.[96,97] Similarly, in Alzheimer disease, patients may have less ability to discriminate between odors or to properly identify them.[98,99]

## Psychiatric Disorders (Depression or Anxiety) and Loss of Smell

Although psychiatric disorders may occur in conjunction with smell dysfunction, having a smell disturbance may lead to depression or anxiety in social situations. It is important to distinguish organic psychiatric disorders from malingerers; the former may have an olfactory loss and have related anxiety or depression or social stigmatizing secondarily, whereas the latter are merely seeking financial or psychological gains. Be aware of patients who exaggerate taste and/or smell loss while failing to mention smoking and medical comorbidities that may affect their smell dysfunction.[100]

## Common Causes of Taste Loss or Distortion (Rarer)

Most of this article addresses olfactory disturbances, which are common, whereas true organic taste disturbances are unusual. There are several common causes of taste loss.

## Olfactory loss (perceived taste loss)

Most patients who complain of a taste loss suffer from an olfactory deficit. The duality of flavor speaks to this process. Olfactory losses that are perceived as taste loss by the patients typically present with the inability to perceive complex flavors of food/beverages but they still retain the function of taste perception of bitter, salty, sour, sweet, and umami.[101] The best method of determining an olfactory loss is with testing. The facial plastic surgeon should recognize this association.

## Medications

Many medications can alter or decrease both taste and smell perception (**Table 3**).[102]

## Infection (fungal thrush, bacterial, viral, URI, parasitic) and mucositis (after radiation)

Oral infections such as fungal thrush, bacterial pharyngitis, viral/URI, and parasitic infections all affect taste to some degree. Inflammatory mediators and direct injury to tissue and taste papillae from pathogen invasion and associated cytokine response may temporarily alter taste. Conversely, patients who undergo radiation to the salivary glands or oral cavity often experience mucositis and decreased taste sensation. To some degree, artificial saliva and hydration alleviate the discomfort but may not assist with taste perception.

## Neoplasm

It is well established that a neoplasm, especially in the floor of the mouth or tongue can alter taste. In addition, both glossectomy and oral cavity resections distort anatomy. Smoking or chewing tobacco may cause dysgeusia/hypogeusia mediated through direct toxic injury[102] as well as secondary free radicals.

## Poor oral hygiene

Odontogenic infections and dental caries also contribute to altered taste sensations.

## Chorda tympani injury

As previously described, cranial nerve VII via the chorda tympani relates taste perception from the anterior two-thirds of the tongue. If there is a temporal bone tumor, infection, or history of otologic surgery, the chorda may be injured, altering a patient's taste. Likewise, injury to the glossopharyngeal nerve is a known complication after tonsillectomy. These patients generally regain taste sensation within 1 month.

## Age-related alterations (decrease in bitterness or sour)

In the elderly, the taste threshold can be more than twice as high as that of the general population, and drugs and disease states may further decrease taste.[103]

## Toxins (smoking)

Multiple toxins exist in our environment that may be inhaled, ingested, or absorbed systemically, and are associated with dysgeusia. **Table 2** lists various such substances.

## Systemic diseases (burning mouth or Sjogren syndrome)

Systemic diseases affect taste more readily than olfaction. However, the mechanism remains unclear.

**Table 3**
**Medicines that can affect taste and smell**

| Drugs That May Affect Taste and Smell | |
| --- | --- |
| Classification | Drug(s) |
| Amebicides and anthelmintics | Metronidazole, niridazole |
| Anesthetics, local | Benzocaine, procaine hydrochloride (Novocain) and others, cocaine hydrochloride, tetracaine hydrochloride |
| Antilipemic agents | Clofibrate |
| Anticoagulants | Phenindione |
| Anticonvulsants | Lamotrigine |
| Antihistamines | Chlorpheniramine maleate |
| Antimicrobial agents | Amphotericin B, ampicillin, cefamandole, griseofulvin, ethambutol hydrochloride, lincomycin, protease inhibitors, sulfasalazine, sulfones, streptomycin, terbinafine, tetracyclines, tyrothricin |
| Antiproliferative, including immunosuppressive agents | Doxorubicin and methotrexate, azathioprine, carmustine, vincristine sulfate |
| Antirheumatic, analgesic-antipyretic, antiinflammatory agents | Allopurinol, colchicine, gold, levamisole, D-penicillamine, phenylbutazone, 5-thiopyriodoxine |
| Antiseptics | Hexetidine |
| Antithyroid agents | Carbimazole, methimazole, methylthiouracil, propylthiouracil, thiouracil |
| Agents for dental hygiene | Sodium lauryl sulfate (toothpaste) |
| Calcium channel blockers | Nifedipine, diltiazem |
| Diuretics and antihypertensive agents | Captopril, diazoxide, ethacrynic acid, losartan |
| Hypoglycemic drugs | Glipizide, phenformin, and derivatives |
| Muscle relaxants and drugs for treatment of Parkinson disease | Baclofen, chlormezanone, L-dopa |
| Opiates | Codeine, hydromorphone hydrochloride, morphine |
| Psychopharmacologic, including antiepileptic drugs | Carbamazepine, lithium carbonate, phenytoin, psilocybin, trifluoperazine |
| Sympathomimetic drugs | Amphetamines, phenmetrazine theoclate and fenbutrazate hydrochloride (combined) |
| Vasodilators | Oxyfedrine, bamifylline hydrochloride |
| Others | Germine monoacetate, hydroquinone, idoxuridine, iron sorbitex, vitamin D, industrial chemicals (including insecticides), smokeless tobacco, sumatriptan nasal spray |

Data from Schiffman SS. Taste and smell in disease. N Engl J Med 1983;308:1275.

Sjogren syndrome and rheumatoid arthritis are intimately associated with gustatory dysfunction. Another syndrome associated with taste disturbances is burning mouth syndrome (burning pain, dysgeusia and dysesthesia, parasthesia, ageusia). Patients report a metallic or diminished taste. A recent study in California recognized an association with female sex and age more than 30 years.[104]

This review recommended treatment to suppress neurologic function to alleviate pain.

## TREATMENT OF OLFACTORY LOSS

A patient's quality of life is affected after an olfactory loss, from enjoying a meal to safety around toxic chemicals. However, olfactory losses are often irreversible and lack proven therapeutic treatments. Determining the cause of the olfactory deficit is imperative in counseling the patient and predicting the likelihood of improvement. Sensorineural losses are less likely to recover, whereas conductive losses, for example obstructive nasal polyps, are more easily treatable.

Conductive smell losses resulting in hyposmia or anosmia after nasal surgery or obstructing URIs have treatments available. Nasal treatments, including saline irrigations and a nasal steroid spray, may decrease nasal membrane edema, increase nasal airflow, and improve olfaction. Likewise, if the olfactory cleft is obstructed by polyps or tumor or viral inflammation, then surgical excision may be of benefit. Medicines such as high dose oral steroid boluses tapered over 3 weeks have been studied with promising results.[86] A recent study noted that a systemic steroid administration is useful in distinguishing between a conductive loss that will improve and a sensorineural loss that will not respond.[105] Other antiinflammatory or antihistamine medications are also beneficial. A superimposed bacterial infection may be present and a course of antibiotics will restore olfaction. In select circumstances, the patient may have a small amount of residual olfaction that needs to be retrained. In this case, instructing the patients to train their sense of smell with spices is helpful. Again, nasal hygiene and supportive saline mists, humidity, and irrigations will not harm the patient and may be of benefit.

For sensorineural olfactory losses, no proven treatments exist. These losses include age-related loss and congenital loss. A recent study of the use of minocycline as an antiapoptotic agent in patients with postinfectious anosmia and hyposmia found that the patients' olfactory ability after a 2-week course showed no difference whether they took placebo or minocycline.[59]

Olfactory distortions (parosmias and phantosmias) typically resolve in 11 months.[106] Treatments that may be helpful in the interim include occluding the nostril or neuropathic medications such as gabapentin. Anticonvulsants such as Lyrica (pregabalin) also have some success. There is hope for these patients, many of whom are depressed with the perceived hopelessness of their condition. Treatments for hypogeusia or ageusia remain of negligible benefit because there are no effective therapies for taste loss. Again, most true taste loss is medication related and, by changing medicines and discontinuing others, the astute physician may identify the offending agent. Adjunctive to this treatment are local tongue medicines such as steroid creams, artificial saliva, and viscous lidocaine preparations. If the hypogeusia is related to a tumor diagnosis, biopsy with appropriate oncologic treatment is paramount. Dental hygiene and treating periodontal disease may assist in perceived taste disturbances. Often, taste disturbances that coincide with a systemic disease, such as rheumatoid arthritis or Sjogren syndrome, are chronic alterations but may dissipate with control and treatment of the systemic disease. Zinc administered orally has shown benefit in several studies and may be a suitable treatment alternative.[107]

## Quality of Life with Olfactory Loss

Quality of life remains at the forefront of these patients' minds because olfaction gives them the ability to appreciate foods, flavor, and so forth. In this respect, training the hyposmic or anosmic patient to appreciate remaining sensory modalities such as texture of food, pungency, residual taste, and mouth feel is beneficial. In addition, in patients with hypsomia, there is value in training the patient to think about the proximity of the smell and intensifying the smell by bringing it closer.[108] Likewise, encouraging patients to increase food options and trials of different foods is warranted. Adding hot sauces or Asian or ethnic foods may better stimulate the trigeminal nerve promoting sensation.

Protection remains a critical aspect of smell loss. Educating patients' family members so that they are able to inform the patient if the cheese in the refrigerator smells foul or not to consume the spoiled milk is paramount from a safety standpoint. Patients with olfactory loss must use smoke and natural gas detectors in their homes and offices. Converting to an electric powered system may be safer.[108] The physician should counsel the patients regarding the necessity of these items. If the patient lives alone, it is particularly important to use proper refrigeration and storage techniques, use thermometers when cooking, refer to expiration dates, and label older foods. Regular home inspections may be useful. In social situations, having a confidant who the patient can trust to indicate whether cologne or other odors are too strong is helpful as well.[108]

## FUTURE IMPLICATIONS FOR OLFACTION LOSS

Much is known about the link between neurodegenerative disorders and olfaction, and this relationship may one day serve as a screening tool or early diagnostic test Alzheimer disease or Parkinson disease. The pathophysiology is still being investigated. Nonetheless, the senses of taste and smell offer unique opportunities in diagnosis and treatment of neurocognitive conditions and obesity-related ingestive behaviors.

## IN SUMMARY: OLFACTION AND TASTE

Olfaction and taste promote satisfaction and protection in daily life. The astute facial plastic surgeon recognizes the importance of establishing a baseline smell test to document the patients' olfactory status before surgery. After surgery, the surgeon must be alert to the possible mechanisms of hyposmia and anosmia and the pertinent treatment strategies. The surgeon must also understand the importance of counseling the patient and family regarding the cause of the dysfunction and the proper treatments. However, reliable treatments are primarily only available for conductive olfactory losses today. Further research is being conducted to determine the involvement of the olfactory neuron in disease and perhaps, in the future, medicine will discover how to restore a damaged sense of smell.

## REFERENCES

1. Kimmelman CP. The risk to olfaction from nasal surgery. Laryngoscope 1994;104:981–8.
2. Miman MC, Mehmet K, Altuntas A, et al. How smell tests experience and education affect ENT specialists' attitudes towards smell disorders? A survey study. Eur Arch Otorhinolaryngol 2011;268(5):691–4.
3. Hoogland PV, van den Berg R, Huisman E. Misrouted olfactory fibers and ectopic olfactory glomeruli in normal humans and in Parkinson and Alzheimer patients. Neuropathol Appl Neurobiol 2003;29:303–11.
4. Holbrook E, Leopold DA. Physiology of olfaction. In: Flint PW, Haughey BH, Lund VJ, et al, editors. Cummings otolaryngology head and neck surgery. 5th edition. Philadelphia: Mosby; 2010. chapter 41.
5. Mosby's medical dictionary. 8th edition. Elsevier; 2009.
6. Cullen MM, Leopold DA. Disorders of smell and taste. Med Clin North Am 1999;83:57–74.
7. Jafek BW. Ultrastructure of human nasal mucosa. Laryngoscope 1983;93:1576.
8. Stern K, McClintock MK. Regulation of ovulation by human pheromones. Nature 1998;392:177–9.
9. Berliner DL, MontiBloch L, Jennings-White C, et al. The functionality of the human vomeronasal organ (VNO): evidence for steroid receptors. Steroid Biochem Mol Biol 1996;58:259.
10. Keverne EB. The vomeronasal organ. Science 1999;286(5440):716–20.
11. Moran DT, Rowley JC III, Jafek BW. Electron microscopy of human olfactory epithelium reveals a new cell type: the microvillar cell. Brain Res 1982;253:39.
12. Moran DT, Rowley JC 3rd, Jafek BW, et al. The fine structure of the olfactory mucosa in man. J Neurocytol 1982;11:721.
13. Morrison EE, Costanzo RM. Morphology of the human olfactory epithelium. J Comp Neurol 1990;297:1.
14. Rowley JC III, Moran DT, Jafek BW. Peroxidase backfills suggest the mammalian olfactory epithelium contains a second morphologically distinct class of bipolar sensory neuron: the microvillar cell. Brain Res 1989;502:387.
15. Zou Z, Li F, Buck LB. Odor maps in the olfactory cortex. Proc Natl Acad Sci U S A 2005;102(21):7724–9.
16. Laffort P, Patte F, Etcheto M. Olfactory coding on the basis of physiochemical properties. Ann N Y Acad Sci 1974;237:193.
17. Standring S, editor. Gray's anatomy. 40th edition. Philadelphia: Churchill Livingstone (Elsevier); 2008. ch. 30 Oral Cavity. p. 507.
18. Chilfala WM, Polzella DJ. Smell and taste classification of the same stimuli. J Gen Psychol 1995;122:287.
19. Sakai N, Kobayakawa T, Gotow N, et al. Enhancement of sweetness ratings of aspartame by a vanilla odor presented either by orthonasal or retronasal routes. Percept Mot Skills 2001;92(3):1002.
20. Burdach KJ, Doty RL. The effects of mouth movements, swallowing, and spitting on retronasal odor perception. Physiol Behav 1987;41:353.
21. Mozell MM, Stern NM, Mozell MM, et al. Reversal of hyposmia in laryngectomized patients. Chem Senses 1986;11:397.
22. Firestein S. How the olfactory system makes sense of scents. Nature 2001;413:211.
23. Engen T. The perception of odors. New York: Academic Press; 1982.
24. Herz RS, Cupchik GC. The emotional distinctiveness of odor-evoked memories. Chem Senses 1995;20:517.
25. Wippich W, Mecklenbrauker S, Trouet J. Implicit and explicit memories of odors. Arch Psychol (Frankf) 1989;141:195 [in German].
26. Gaillard D, Passilly-Degrace P, Besnard P. Molecular mechanisms of fat preference and overeating. Ann N Y Acad Sci 2008;1141:163–75.
27. Hofer D, Asan E, Drenckhahn D. Chemosensory perception in the gut. News Physiol Sci 1999;14:18–23.
28. Khan NA, Besnard P. Oro-sensory perception of dietary lipids: new insights into the fat taste transduction. Biochim Biophys Acta 2009;1791:149–55.
29. Laugerette F, Passilly-Degrace P, Patris B, et al. CD36 involvement in orosensory detection of dietary lipids, spontaneous fat preference, and digestive secretions. J Clin Invest 2005;115:3177–84.

30. Zhang XJ, Zhou LH, Ban X, et al. Decreased expression of CD36 in circumvallate taste buds of high-fat diet induced obese rats. Acta Histochem 2011; 113(6):663–7. DOI:10.1016/j.acthis.2010.09.007.

31. Estrem SA, Renner G. Disorders of smell and taste. Otolaryngol Clin North Am 1987;20:133–47.

32. Landis BN, Konnerth CG, Hummel T. A study on the frequency of olfactory dysfunction. Laryngoscope 2004;114:1764–9.

33. Cain WS, Gent JF, Goodspeed RB, et al. Evaluation of olfactory dysfunction in the Connecticut Chemosensory Clinical Research Center. Laryngoscope 1988;98:83.

34. Davidson TM, Murphy C. Rapid clinical evaluation of anosmia: the alcohol sniff test. Arch Otolaryngol Head Neck Surg 1997;123:591.

35. Cornsweet TN. The staircase method in psychophysics. Am J Psychol 1962;75:485.

36. Levitt H. Transformed up-down methods in psychophysics. J Acoust Soc Am 1971;49:467.

37. Heywood PG, Costanzo RM. Identifying normosmics: a comparison of two populations. Am J Otolaryngol 1986;7:194.

38. Punter PH. Measurements of human olfactory thresholds for several groups of structurally related compounds. Chem Senses 1983;7:215.

39. MacKay-Sim A, Doty RL. University of Pennsylvania smell identification test: normative adjustment for Australian subjects. Aust J Otolaryngol 2001.

40. Doty RL, Shaman P, Dann M. Development of the University of Pennsylvania Smell Identification Test: a standardized microencapsulated test of olfactory function. Physiol Behav 1984;32:489.

41. Doty RL, Shaman P, Kimmelman CP, et al. University of Pennsylvania Smell Identification Test: a rapid quantitative olfactory function test for the clinic. Laryngoscope 1984;94:176.

42. Tagagi SF. A standardized olfactometer in Japan. Ann N Y Acad Sci 1987;510:113.

43. Wolfensberger M, Schnieper I, Welge-Lussen A. Sniffin' Sticks: a new olfactory test battery. Acta Otolaryngol 2000;120:303.

44. Klingmuller D, Dewes W, Krahe T, et al. Magnetic resonance imaging of the brain in patients with anosmia and hypothalamic hypogonadism (Kallmann's syndrome). J Clin Endocrinol Metab 1987; 65:581.

45. Li C, Yousem DM, Doty RL, et al. Neuroimaging in patients with olfactory dysfunction. AJR Am J Roentgenol 1994;162:411.

46. Suzuki M, Takashima T, Kadoya M, et al. MR imaging of olfactory bulbs and tracts. AJNR Am J Neuroradiol 1989;10:955.

47. Pasquale F, Finelli PF, Mair RG. Disturbances of smell and taste. ch. 19. In: Bradley, editor. neurology in clinical practice. 5th edition. Philadelphia (PA): Butterworth-Heinemann; 2008. p. 256–7, 260.

48. Kern RC. Chronic sinusitis and anosmia: pathologic changes in the olfactory mucosa. Laryngoscope 2000;110:1071.

49. Kern RC, Conley DB, Haines GK 3rd, et al. Pathology of the olfactory mucosa: implications for the treatment of olfactory dysfunction. Laryngoscope 2004;114:279–85.

50. Hendriks AP. Olfactory dysfunction. Rhinology 1988;26:229.

51. Akerlund A, Bende M, Murphy C. Olfactory threshold and nasal mucosal changes in experimentally induced common cold. Acta Otolaryngol 1995;115:88.

52. Jafek BW, Hartman D, Eller PM, et al. Postviral olfactory dysfunction. Am J Rhinol 1990;4:91–100.

53. Yamagishi M, Fujiwara M, Nakamura H. Olfactory mucosal findings and clinical course in patients with olfactory disorders following upper respiratory viral infection. Rhinology 1994;32:113.

54. Yamagishi M, Hasegawa S, Nakano Y. Examination and classification of human olfactory mucosa in patients with clinical olfactory disturbances. Arch Otorhinolaryngol 1988;245:316.

55. Leopold DA. The relationship between nasal anatomy and human olfaction. Laryngoscope 1988;98:1232.

56. Davidson TM, Jalowayski A, Murphy C, et al. Evaluation and treatment of smell dysfunction. West J Med 1987;146:434.

57. Goodspeed RB, Gent JF, Catalanotto FA. Chemosensory dysfunction: clinical evaluation results from a taste and smell clinic. Postgrad Med 1987; 81:251.

58. Leopold DA, Hornung DE, Youngentob SL. Olfactory loss after upper respiratory infection. In: Getchell T, Bartoshuk LM, Doty RL, et al, editors. Smell and taste in health and disease. New York: Raven Press; 1991. p. 731–4.

59. Reden J, Herting B, Lill K, et al. Treatment of post-infectious olfactory disorders with minocycline: a double-blind, placebo-controlled study. Laryngoscope 2011;121:679–82.

60. Leigh AD. Defect of smell after head injury. Lancet 1943;1:38.

61. Hughes B. The results of injury to special parts of the brain and skull. In: Rowbottom GF, editor. Acute injuries to the head. 4th edition. London: Churchill Livingstone; 1964. p. 277–80.

62. Sumner D. Post-traumatic anosmia. Brain 1964; 87:107.

63. Zusho H. Post-traumatic anosmia. Arch Otolaryngol 1982;108:90.

64. Henkin RI, Schecter PJ, Friedewald WT, et al. A double-blind study of the effects of zinc sulfate on taste and smell dysfunction. Am J Med Sci 1976;272:285.

65. Reiter ER, DiNardo LJ, Costanzo RM. Effects of head injury on olfaction and taste. Otolaryngol Clin North Am 2004;37(6):1167–84.

66. Stevens JC, Cain WS. Old-age deficits in the sense of smell as gauged by thresholds, magnitude matching, and odor identification. Psychol Aging 1987;2:36.

67. Doty RL, Shaman P, Applebaum SL, et al. Smell identification ability: changes with age. Science 1984;226:1441.

68. Liss L, Gomez F. The nature of senile changes of the human olfactory bulb and tract. Arch Otolaryngol 1958;67:167.

69. Jafek BW, Gordon AS, Moran DT, et al. Congenital anosmia. Ear Nose Throat J 1990;69:331.

70. Kallman FJ, Schoenfeld WA, Barrera SE. The genetic aspects of primary eunuchoidism. Am J Ment Defic 1944;48:203.

71. Kanai T. Ober das Kombunerte Verkommen des partieller Reichlappendefecies met dem Eunuchoidismus. Okajimas Folia Anat Jap 1940;19:200 [in German].

72. de Morsier G. La dysplasie olfactogenitale. Acta Neuropathol 1962;1:433 [in French].

73. Dewes W, Krahe T, Klingmüller D, et al. MR tomography of Kallmann's syndrome. Rofo 1987;147:400 [in German].

74. Schwob JE, Szumowski KE, Leopold DA, et al. Histopathology of olfactory mucosa in Kallmann's syndrome. Ann Otol Rhinol Laryngol 1993;102:117.

75. Upadhyay UD, Holbrook EH. Olfactory loss as a result of toxic exposure. Otolaryngol Clin North Am 2004;37:1185–207.

76. Smith DV, Duncan HJ. Primary olfactory disorders: anosmia, hyposmia, and dysosmia. In: Serby MJ, Chobor KL, editors. Science of olfaction. 1st edition. New York: Springer-Verlag; 1992. p. 439–66.

77. Skolnik EM, Massari FS, Fenta LT. Olfactory neuroepithelioma: review of world literature and presentation of two cases. Arch Otolaryngol 1966;84:644.

78. Furstenberg AC, Crosby E, Farrior B. Neurologic lesions which influence the sense of smell. Arch Otolaryngol 1943;48:529.

79. Landis BN, Hummel T, Lacroix JS. Basic and clinical aspects of olfaction. Adv Tech Stand Neurosurg 2005;30:69–105.

80. Henkin RI. Olfaction in human disease. In: English GM, editor. Otolaryngology. New York: Harper and Row; 1982. p. 1–39.

81. Adelman BT. Altered taste and smell after anesthesia: cause and effect? Anesthesiology 1995;83:647–9.

82. Biedlingmaier JF, Whelan P, Zoarski G, et al. Histopathology and CT analysis of partially resected middle turbinates. Laryngoscope 1996;106:102–4.

83. Wigand ME. Endoscopic surgery of the paranasal sinuses and anterior skull base. New York: Thieme Medical Publishers; 1990. p. 134–41.

84. Rettinger G, Kirshe H. Complications in septoplasty. Facial Plast Surg 2006;22(4):289–97.

85. Briner HR, Simmen D, Jones N. Impaired sense of smell in patients with nasal surgery. Clin Otolaryngol Allied Sci 2003;28:417–9.

86. Pade J, Hummel T. Olfactory function following nasal surgery. Laryngoscope 2008;118:1260–4.

87. Champion R. Anosmia associated with corrective rhinoplasty. Br J Plast Surg 1966;19(2):182–5.

88. Goldwyn RM, Shore S. The effects of submucous resection and rhinoplasty on the sense of smell. Plast Reconstr Surg 1968;41:427.

89. Sailer HF, Landolt AM. A new method for the correction of hypertelorism with preservation of the olfactory nerve filaments. J Craniomaxillofac Surg 1987;15:122.

90. Spetzler RF, Herman JM, Beals S, et al. Preservation of olfaction in anterior craniofacial approaches. J Neurosurg 1993;79:48.

91. Tigliev GS, Ilias MI, Dubikaitis IUV. Approach to tumors of the chiasm-sellar region with preservation of the olfactory tracts. Zh Vopr Neirokhir Im N N Burdenko 1986;6:13 [in Russian].

92. Hilgers FJ, van Dam FS, Keyzers S, et al. Rehabilitation of olfaction after laryngectomy by means of a nasal airflow-inducing maneuver: the "polite yawning" technique. Arch Otolaryngol Head Neck Surg 2000;126(6):726–32.

93. Haxel BR, Fuch C, Fruth WJ, et al. Evaluation of the efficacy of the 'nasal airflow-inducing manoeuvre' for smell rehabilitation in laryngectomees by means of the Sniffin' Sticks test. Clin Otolaryngol 2011;36(1):17–23.

94. Berendse HW, Ponsen MM. Detection of preclinical Parkinson's disease along the olfactory trac(t). J Neural Transm Suppl 2006;(70):321–5.

95. Haehner A, Hummel T, Hummel C, et al. Olfactory loss may be first sign of idiopathic Parkinson's disease. Mov Disord 2007;22:839–42.

96. Doty RL, Bromley SM, Stern MB. Olfactory testing as an aid in the diagnosis of Parkinson's disease: development of optimal discrimination criteria. Neurodegeneration 1995;4:93–7.

97. Hummel T, Witt M, Reichmann H, et al. Immunohistochemical, volumetric, and functional neuroimaging studies in patients with idiopathic Parkinson's disease. J Neurol Sci 2010;289:119–22.

98. Morgan CD, Nordin S, Murphy C. Odor identification as an early marker for Alzheimer's disease: impact of lexical functioning and detection sensitivity. J Clin Exp Neuropsychol 1995;17:793–803.

99. Suzuki Y, Yamamoto S, Umegaki H, et al. Smell identification test as an indicator for cognitive impairment. Int J Geriatr Psychiatry 2004;19:727–33.

100. Doty RL, Crastnopol B. Correlates of chemosensory malingering. Laryngoscope 2010;120:707–11.
101. Soter A, Kim J, Jackman A, et al. Accuracy of reporting taste loss is poor. Laryngoscope 2008;118(4):611–7.
102. Finelli PF, Mair RG. Bradley. In: Bradley WG, Daroff RB, Fenichel GM, et al, editors. Neurology in Clinical Practice. 5th edition. Philadelphia (PA): Mosby; 2008. p. 260–2. [Chapter: 19].
103. Schiffman SS. Taste and smell losses in normal aging and disease. JAMA 1997;278:1357–62.
104. Suarez P, Clark GT. Burning mouth syndrome: an update on diagnosis and treatment methods. J Calif Dent Assoc 2006;34(8):611–22.
105. Seiden AM, Duncan HJ. The diagnosis of a conductive olfactory loss. Laryngoscope 2001;111:9–14.
106. Duncan HJ, Seiden AM. Long-term follow-up of olfactory loss secondary to head trauma and upper respiratory tract infection. Arch Otolaryngol Head Neck Surg 1995;121:1183–7.
107. Schecter PJ, Friedewald WT, Bronzert OA, et al. Idiopathic hypogeusia: a description of the syndrome and a single-blind study with zinc sulfate. Int Rev Neurobiol 1972;1:125.
108. Cain WS, Turk A. Smell of danger: an analysis of LP-gas odorization. Am Ind Hyg Assoc J 1985;46:115.

# Index

*Note:* Page numbers of article titles are in **boldface** type.

## A

*N*-Acetylcysteine
  in rhinology, 76, 78
Acupuncture
  in rhinology, 78
Acute rhinosinusitis (ARS)
  CRS and
    microbiology of
      differences in, 88
    MRSA in, 89
Acute sinusitis
  treatment of
    pharmacotherapy in, 66–67
Aging
  loss of taste related to, 105
  olfactory loss related to, 102
Air inspiration
  unified airway and, 58
Airway(s)
  unified, **55–60**. *See also* Unified airway
Airway disease
  clinical
    pathophysiologic mechanisms in, 56–57
Alcohol pad test
  in olfactory and taste disorders, 98
Aller-7
  in rhinology, 78
Allergic diseases. *See also specific diseases*
  pathophysiologic mechanisms in, 56–57
Allergic rhinitis, **11–20**
  asthma and
    relationship between, 56
  concurrent FESS and rhinoplasty for, 46–48
  defined, 11–12
  diagnosis of, 13–16
    challenge testing in, 14–15
    patient history in, 13–14
    physical findings in, 14
    sIgE testing in, 15
    skin testing in, 15
    testing in, 14
    total IgE testing in, 15
  epidemiology of, 12–13
  genetics of, 11–12
  NAR and
    similarities between, 21
  treatment of, 16–18
    antihistamines in, 64–65
    combination therapy in, 66

decongestants in, 65
environmental control in, 16–17
immunotherapy in, 17–18, 66
intranasal anticholinergics in, 65
intranasal corticosteroids in, 64
intranasal cromolyn in, 65
leukotriene receptor antagonists in, 65–66
pharmacotherapy in, 16, 63–66
surgery in, 17
Allergic rhinoconjunctivitis (ARC)
  pathophysiology of, 61–62
  prevalence of, 61
Allergic skin disease, **31–42**. *See also* Atopic dermatitis; Contact dermatitis
Allergy(ies)
  in atopic dermatitis, 35
  CRS due to, 2
  immunology of, 12
Alternative medicine
  described, 73–74
  in rhinology, **73–81**. *See also* Complementary and alternative medicine (CAM), in rhinology
Anatomic factors
  CRS due to, 3
Anesthesia/anesthetics
  topical
    contact dermatitis due to, 38
Angelica
  in rhinology, 76, 78
Antibiotic(s)
  oral
    in CRS management, 5
  topical
    in CRS management, 6
Antibiotic resistance
  in CRS, **87–91**
Anticholinergic(s)
  intranasal
    in allergic rhinitis management, 65
Anticholinergic nasal spray
  in NAR management, 26
Antihistamines
  in allergic rhinitis management, 64–65
  in NAR management, 26
Anxiety
  loss of smell related to, 105
ARC. *See* Allergic rhinoconjunctivitis (ARC)
ARS. *See* Acute rhinosinusitis (ARS)
Ascorbic acid

Facial Plast Surg Clin N Am 20 (2012) 113–118
doi:10.1016/S1064-7406(11)00206-9
1064-7406/12/$ – see front matter © 2012 Elsevier Inc. All rights reserved.

Printed and bound by CPI Group (UK) Ltd, Croydon, CR0 4YY

03/10/2024

01040358-0003